ENLIGHTENED
NUTRITION

Discovering Your Own Ultimate Diet
For Health, Longevity, and Consciousness

PAUL DUGLISS, M.D.

No part of this book is intended to substitute for medical advice, diagnosis, or treatment. Every individual is unique, and no book can possibly address each person's special situation. Do not make changes in your medications or lifestyle without consulting your health care provider. The information contained in this book is intended to stimulate discussion with your health care providers and not to replace their advice.

Cover Design: Ko Wicke – Proglyphics.com

ISBN 978-0-9721233-8-9

This book is dedicated to your health.

ACKNOWLEDGEMENTS

First and foremost, I would like to acknowledge my friend, Sue Niedzielski, without whose support this book would never have been published. I would also like to acknowledge my colleagues Sandra Moss, Aparna Khanolkar, and Jennifer Smith. Without their enthusiasm, persistence, and assistance I would never have completed this book. I would also like to thank them for their contributions to the writing itself. I feel it appropriate also to acknowledge the many teachers that have enabled me to have a life dedicated to medicine and healing, especially Clinton Greenstone, M.D., D. Edwards Smith, M.D., David McClanahan, and Philip Conran.

This book draws on principles that are common to many ancient medical systems. The concepts and method of presenting them is based on my experience teaching patients about diet — a process that continues to be refined. Thus, I must finally acknowledge my patients, who teach me more than I teach them.

– Paul Dugliss, M.D.

CONTENTS

* 1 *

Introduction

We are spiritual beings having a human experience.
— *Teilhard De Chardin*

This book is about you. It is about your experience, your health, and your life. For any topic to be "enlightened," it must contain truth. This book is about *your* truth. It is designed to honor that truth and help you to recognize and value it. While some expert opinion will be presented, along with some advice from thousands of years of dietary knowledge, these are not important. They will only serve to supplement your experience and your discoveries.

This is not a textbook. This is a guidebook. Through the exercises presented here, your experience will guide you to finding the ultimate diet *for you*. Finding that diet is crucial. It determines your future health, your well-being, and your happiness.

Enlightened Nutrition is not about dieting, but it will help you to achieve your optimal weight. It is not about restricting what you eat, but it will help you to choose foods wisely. It is not about denying yourself the pleasure of eating. In fact, it will help you to enjoy eating even more.

This book is about you because it is about how you can rediscover the truth about diet and health and what is best for your particular physiology. Whether your interest is weight loss, weight gain, food allergies, or perfect health, reading about diet is too often inadequate. Experiencing the benefits of your ultimate diet is the only meaningful way for dietary change to be lasting. That fact compels this book to be different from other books on diet.

Each section of the book will be based on some experience you have had, or are willing to try to have. Each principle will be a principle you can verify yourself. Your experience and the experience of hundreds of others like you form the basis for the principles of Enlightened Nutrition.

My hope is that this new approach to verifying the wisdom of the ancients will propel you to new heights of awareness and well-being. Health, ultimately, is about experiencing wholeness, not about restriction and discipline. Experiencing that complete wholeness called perfect health and discovering your own ultimate diet is my goal for each person who reads this book.

* 2 *

Rediscovering Truth

Time's glory is to calm contending kings,
To unmask falsehood, and bring truth to light.
— *Shakespeare*

When it comes to the discussion of diet, truth is hard to find. Just like a political or religious debate, the subject is emotionally charged. Opinions abound. Many "experts" offer rational explanations why one should eat this way or that way. Just go to any bookstore and search for books on diet and health. You will find a vast array, all touting good reasons why you should adopt their diets. Which one is right for you?

Each book focuses on getting us to try its diet. Somewhere inside of us, we resist doing that. Why? Perhaps because it is not *our* diet, it is *their* diet. Even when we know some change is in order, the fact that someone else who doesn't know us is making up rules and guidelines for us creates some resistance. Aren't we each unique? How do we know that this diet is right for us?

As a health care provider, I see the impact diet has on people's lives every day. I have seen people advised and cajoled, researched and lectured, admonished and praised, and still I find that dietary change is hard to achieve. I have seen the impact of what happens when dietary guidelines come from "the outside." I have seen what happens when "the experts" make recommendations. I have researched the ancient wisdom from the Vedic tradition of India to the wisdom of Chinese Medicine and ancient Japanese knowledge and have presented this to hundreds of patients in patient education classes. I have presented modern medical research supporting the ancient traditions. Still, dietary changes came slowly, until I realized the importance of *experiencing* the truth.

Why publish another book on diet? Because this book will guide you to experience the fundamental truths surrounding diet and health. This book will help you to verify the wisdom of the ancients. It is this different approach that motivates yet another book on diet.

One other reason motivates the writing of this book. Your health. Regardless of the huge sums of money that are spent on health care in the United States, health is not breaking out all over. Although our understanding of biology, genetics, and medical technology has become increasingly advanced, we are not healthier. In 1990, the Assistant Dean of Medical Education at the Medical College of Ohio informed my class that, by the end of the decade, we would have spent more than 1.2 trillion dollars on diseases that were entirely preventable. That decade has come and gone, and more than that amount was spent on preventable diseases. The key ingredient in most of the prevention strategies that could have succeeded? Diet.

All sorts of documentation is currently available showing that medical science has proved the importance of diet and its potency in preventing disease. Thousands of research studies have been published. In spite of all this knowledge, modern medicine is still focused on drugs, not on diet — on disease management, not on prevention.

What is the key element missing in diet books, in modern medical research, and in fad diets? A means to help people change and a means to experience firsthand the principles that guide a healthy diet — these are what have been missing. The truth I am speaking about is the truth about how nature works.

This book is about rediscovering truth. It is about personal truth. It is about *your* truth. It is about rediscovering the ancient truths in your own awareness and own experience. After much experience and experimentation, this seems to be the best means I have found for achieving lasting change. Diet fads come and go, but what you experience and integrate as your own personal knowledge stays with you forever. I am not the first to find that the laws of nature that govern the functioning of the body can be known firsthand.

History records that many of the great cultures of ancient times had seers or sages who sat together to explore how nature works. Part of this exploration was rediscovering how diet and health are related. These explorations can be found in the ancient medical traditions of India, China, Tibet, and Japan. These predictable principles were called "natural law" because, like laws of physics, they were consistent and verifiable. The seers had much to say about health, and many of their sayings later became canonized into the classical texts of Ayurveda, the ancient healing tradition of India, as well as the classical texts of Chinese Medicine.

Just as physics operates on consistent laws that can be rediscovered, natural laws can also be rediscovered. Natural laws are the complex outcomes that come from the more fundamental laws of physics. Even if we don't know the mathematics that describes the elliptical orbit of the sun, we know that it is a law of nature that spring follows winter. We don't have fall following winter. We don't have summer following winter. While it is not a profound law, it is a natural law that there is an order to the seasons. Natural laws are like this. They describe larger, more complex phenomena that are built on the fundamental laws of physics.

Another example of natural law is that "like increases like." If you take a light, airy individual and feed them a light, airy diet, they lose weight, and that individual's lightness increases. This is an example of a whole series of complex physical and biological laws that comprise what is known as a natural law.

A whole science of the natural laws governing health is known in the East. Natural law in India is known as Veda, and this science of health is called Ayurveda.

THE INSIDE SCOOP

Ayurveda

The word "Ayurveda" comes from two words: "ayur" meaning life or longevity, and "veda" meaning truth, knowledge, or science. Ayurveda then refers to the science of longevity or the truth of life. While it is often considered a system of medicine based on classical texts, its true basis is in "veda" or the truth found in natural law. Just as the laws of physics can be rediscovered and logically deduced, so too, "veda" can be cognized because it is inherent in how nature works.

The ancient sages who cognized the natural laws that make up Ayurveda recognized that there were fundamental laws underlying all of creation (i.e., how creation got created). If you understand the qualities that determine whether a plant, food, herb, or substance is light or airy, heavy or stable, fiery or intense, then you can understand how to use that substance to create balance in the human body.

The compilation of the understanding of these natural laws forms the medicine known as Ayurveda that is the primary care medicine for approximately 800 million people in India and southeast Asia.

In the West, our search for truth has come mainly from looking to the outside. Science is composed of the following:

- *Observations that can be verified.*
- *Experiments that can be replicated.*
- *Conclusions that can be deduced by anyone who is logical.*

Science is a useful tool, but it is not the only tool. You have precious tools for discovering truth and "recognizing" natural law. The only difference between you and the seers is the refined awareness or consciousness that they had developed (something you can develop, too, through the practice of meditation). Because consciousness can vary so much from individual to individual, the need for an objective way of knowing developed. Science has filled that void. The other approach, the subjective approach to knowledge, can be just as valid. The missing variable has been a means to develop consciousness to its full capacity. Even before that, though, your awareness is a valuable tool. With a little guidance, it can be used to rediscover the knowledge of diet and dietary principles cognized by the ancients.

We all have some awareness of our experience. We all have intuition. Each of has a "gut feeling" about what is right for us. Intuition and awareness can be guided and refined to know the most profound principles of diet and health. This book helps you to develop these precious tools.

I invite you to undertake this different approach to diet and dietary principles. I invite you to utilize your awareness and allow that awareness to be guided to discovering what is healthiest for you. As you do so, you will start to experience the fundamental principles of Enlightened Nutrition. Some of these principles you will learn through direct experience, some through others experiences. Each will be supported by some of the cognitions of the ancient seers. Each will be supported by the findings of modern science. In this manner, you will rediscover truth in your own awareness and in your own body.

This process may make for lasting changes in the way you think about diet, the way you eat, the types of things you eat, and ultimately, the way you re-create yourself. My hope is that you will stop thinking of food in terms of nutrients and calories and start thinking of it in terms of energy, qualities, and the spiritual impact it has on human beings. All this radical shift requires is an openness to learn from your experience.

Each of the following chapters is designed to convey one of the fundamental principles of Enlightened Nutrition. Each chapter will start with an experiment or an experience. These experiments will allow you to discover the important principles of diet *before* each principle is presented. Then some of the experiences my patients have had will be presented.

These will help you to be aware of the consistencies in experience. I will then present and discuss the principle *and* its implications in detail. This knowledge will be further verified with some of the sayings of the ancients, as well as some research from modern science. In some cases, further exercises to hone in on the point will be suggested. Further recommendations from the ancient seers will be presented so that you can fully apply the principle in your daily life. Speaking of daily life ... practical recipes based on what you have learned will also be presented.

Now begins a very interesting and enjoyable journey ...

* 3 *

Life Energy

To eat is human. To digest is divine.
— Mark Twain

Tom S. is the third patient of the afternoon with the identical complaint, "I'm constantly tired." Fatigue is probably the second most common complaint in any primary care physician's office. "I have been thinking that I am just getting older, but I want to make sure that is all it is." I tell him fatigue is not a part of aging. I have seen 90-year-olds who have more energy than Tom. As I go through his lifestyle, point by point, two things stand out. Tom has been attempting to maintain a harrowing pace that has been consuming his energy reserves, and his diet has been devoid of anything that would replace those energies. He is puzzled as to his fatigue because he has slowed down his pace for two months and is feeling no better. I asked him to enroll in one of my cooking classes. He does, and from the very first experiment, he knows exactly why he hasn't been able to recover his energies. This experiment is presented for you below.

Writing down your observations helps to deepen the experience and helps you to remember as you analyze some questions I have for you. Caution: Do not try this experiment if you have an ulcer or an allergy to orange juice.

There is no right or wrong experience. What you experience is important – what you feel is real. It is as simple as that. Your experience may differ from others experiences – the reason for that will be explained shortly.

Experiment #1

The Orange Juice Experiment

Required Materials:
1 - 2 fresh juicy organic oranges
1 small carton of room temperature orange juice
2 identical glasses

Method:
1) Pour 1/2 cup of orange juice from the carton into one glass.

2) Slice the 1 - 2 oranges in half, and then squeeze into the other glass until there is exactly the same amount of juice as in the first glass (be sure to filter out any seeds).

3) If possible, go into another room and have someone rotate the glasses several times, so that you won't know which is which.

4) Smell each glass, then pick one and take a sip of it, paying attention to the taste. Then consume the entire glass.

5) Repeat step 4 with the other glass.

6) Write down your reaction to this experience.

Stop!!! If you haven't already done the experiment, now is the time to put the book down, and give it a try.

Here are some questions about this experiment for you to ponder:

1) Is there a difference between the two glasses?

2) How would you describe the difference, if there is one?

3) Why should there be any difference between the two? Let's analyze that last question a bit further. Both glasses contain orange juice. Both juices contain water. Both contain vitamin C. Biochemical analysis would show that they are both the same substance — orange juice. So why would one taste different from the other?

4) How does your body feel after taking the freshly-squeezed orange juice?

5) Based on how your body reacts to the freshly-squeezed orange juice, what might you deduce are the long-term effects of taking foods that are like the carton orange juice?

Not everyone's awareness is developed to the point where they immediately experience the impact of a small amount of food on the body. Still, many people do report some awareness of this impact. It brings out the point that different people have different degrees of awareness. Don't get stressed if you didn't notice much. You will eventually notice more as you pay more attention. Here is what some others have said after trying this experiment. Try to wait to read these until after you have had time to reflect on your own experience.

"I noticed immediately that there was a difference, but I had a hard time putting it into words. The fresh orange juice was definitely more pleasing, and I was attracted to it more, but I was not sure why that would be."
— *Deborah G., Office Manager*

"I could tell a real liveliness to the fresh-squeezed orange juice. The other just fell flat. It felt dull … dead in comparison."
— *James L., Marketing Director*

"To be honest, they tasted pretty much the same to me. Not completely alike, but with the same sweet and sour kind of taste. The taste was more intense maybe … more distinctive with the fresh-squeezed orange juice."
— *Suzanne T., Secretary*

"My experience with tasting the difference between the two was a bit startling. I haven't had much fresh-squeezed orange juice in my life, and compared to that it was like drinking a different fruit juice altogether. The fresh stuff was so tangy and just felt so alive. The carton juice tasted flat and uninteresting. Just a sip of the fresh juice made me feel more alive and awake."
— *Lisa B., Student*

Even though the biochemical makeup of these two juices is the same, the taste for most people is different. Why? The answer to this question can be summed up in two words: *life energy*. Life energy is sometimes called *prana* in the ancient texts of Ayurveda. It is called *chi* in the ancient Chinese texts and *ki* in Traditional Japanese Medicine. *Prana* is sometimes translated as "vital breath" or "breath of life" but goes far beyond the intake of air. It relates to life force or life energy.

For those of you who had difficulty detecting a difference, try repeating the experiment for three or four days in a row, first thing in the morning before eating anything. You will start to notice the difference others describe. Remember that the sages had a means for developing perception and awareness. For them, the influence of a given food could be perceived far into the future. They could tell that by taking certain foods in the summer they would feel warmer in winter. They could tell which tissues in the body were being nourished from foods taken a week or a month earlier.

It takes some time meditating and developing consciousness for most of us to perceive on that level. But for now, we can get a glimpse by doing some of these experiments and recognizing that we may need to repeat the experiment more than once.

The vast majority of people immediately notice a difference, and some sensitive people tend to feel a different impact coming from the fresh-squeezed orange juice. Often difficult to put into words, they describe it as imparting a certain "liveliness" or "freshness." This liveliness relates to the life energy contained in the fresh oranges. It gives rise to our first basic principle or natural law and the logical conclusion you can make from this experience:

Principle #1: Food Conveys Life Energy

Life energy is not the same as calories. Calories give the body "fuel" to burn to keep the body temperature stable. They don't necessarily give the body vitality and liveliness. These qualities are so lacking in the American diet that it is no wonder fatigue is one of the most common complaints in doctors' offices. When fatigue becomes chronic, it is difficult to feel happy. Depression sets in. This common condition is treated with drugs that attempt to supplement the biochemicals the brain should be producing, rather than looking for the underlying source of emotional exhaustion. It is simple logic that if food is devoid of life energy, fatigue and depression will be more likely to take hold.

Food conveys life energy in addition to supplying calories. The more this fresh liveliness is present, the more vital and vibrant the individual. Exist on canned food for several years, and it will not take a psychic to perceive the loss of vibrancy, the dullness in the complexion, the lack of clarity in thinking.

Consider also what the impact might be on the feedback mechanisms in the body. The body's sense of hunger, fullness, and satisfaction is a very fined-tuned mechanism. Being off by only a few calories a day can amount to significant weight gain or weight loss in just one year's time.

What is the impact of taking foods that have sufficient calories but do not supply life energy? This lack of life energy can cause the feedback mechanisms to misread. Because energy is lacking in the food, the body can signal to continue eating when excess calories have already been consumed. I see this as one of the major causes of obesity. Food that is lacking in life energy has no liveliness with which to nourish the mind and emotions. While the body may get excess calories to burn, the person is undernourished. This is starving in the midst of plenty. This is, in part, what motivates excessive eating. You might be surprised to find that overweight people often complain of feeling fatigued. From this perspective, it is no wonder.

THE SCIENCE BEHIND THE SAGES

LIFE ENERGY (PRANA)

This subtle life energy is not usually visible to the naked eye of nonclairvoyant individuals. The best tool to show physical evidence of the life energy in objects is Kirlian photography. Kirlian photography provides indirect electrographic images of the "etheric body" of living and nonliving beings.

The etheric body is a highly structured energy field surrounding our physical body. It functions to provide unique energetic information to the cells of the physical body. It works in concert with unfolding patterns of genetic information. This information is essential to the proper growth and development of the living beings. For further illustration, in his book, *Vibrational Medicine*, Richard Gerber, M.D., explains that the etheric body functions as the invisible scaffolding upon which grow the primitive cells of the developing human fetus.

Clairvoyants report that it serves as an invisible "mold" that subtly guides the process of unfoldment of the fetus' physical form. In the event of physical trauma to our physical body, our etheric body carries the energy template helping to direct the repair and rebuilding. It assists to direct the biochemical and electrical cellular information systems inherent in our physical body. It is believed that "disturbances" and "distorted patterns of energetic information" in the etheric body contribute to the development of disease and illness.

Kirlian photography takes pictures of an object in the presence of a high-frequency electrical field. A power generator produces a high-voltage, high-frequency electrical field that "bathes" the object being electrographically photographed. The object, say a leaf, is in turn highly electrically charged. In the process, a "spark discharge" around the leaf is created. The spark discharge produces light that exposes photographic film on which the object was originally placed. The end product is the capturing of the object's "aura" or a coronal energy discharge.

THE SCIENCE BEHIND THE SAGES (cont.)

It is thought that Kirlian photography records the sum of the electrical potential of cells. The degree of electrical conductivity, in turn, is representative of the energy of the whole system. The strength of the electroluminescence of the Kirlian photography indicates the strength of the life energy of cells. Strong and intact energy fields are able to better maintain the physical structure and function of the system.

Researchers have been able to study how the life force of people and foods is affected by various conditions. The photograph of 12 subjects who were put on a 24-hour diet of junk food revealed an absence of any electroluminescent energy. In contrast, a highly charged field was captured around the body of an individual who had been eating whole foods for 40 years. In another comparison, a photograph was taken of a cabbage before and after being cooked in a pressure cooker for 10 minutes. The raw cabbage had a significantly brighter and larger electroluminescent field than the cooked cabbage.

Food conveys its liveliness to the eater. Vibrant health requires vibrant and lively food. Food that is fresh and freshly prepared *is* different from old, packaged, frozen, canned, and leftover food. What you experience in the orange juice experiment is the subtle difference between the fresh food and old food. What you don't experience is the long-term effects of taking old food, day in and day out.

Food that is full of life energy gives not only vibrant energy to the body, it also gives intelligent energy to the body. Intelligent energy is energy that can help to maintain proper order and functioning in the body. It has its ability to stimulate the body to "remember" the proper functioning. It is said by the ancients that it has the intelligence or "memory value" intact. A useful analogy might be a rocket. You can put a lot of high-energy fuel in the rocket, but without a guidance system, it is likely to end up in the ocean, rather than on the moon. Just like that, food that has lots of *prana* or *chi* brings not only life energy to the body, but also intelligence to its functioning.

What is the end result of a diet completely devoid of "intelligent functioning"? Clearly one result from the perspective of the sages is disordered functioning of cells. When a cell starts to replicate and function in-dependently of its surrounding cells, that functioning is disordered and unintelligent. Eventually this unhindered growth results in the condition called cancer. This is only one example of what happens when a cell loses its "memory" or intelligence value. Many of our modern ills can be traced to this loss of lively intelligence in the body.

At this point, it may seem that I am making a great deal out of a little glass of orange juice. What you experience with your awareness is only one moment of time. You do not experience directly its effects over time without some development of awareness. The difference that you experience has meaning. It has meaning for your body, your health, and your future. When I present this to my patients, few have difficulty understanding that the effect can be subtle and yet significant. I *am* making a big deal out of it, because it *is* a big deal that you experience in a small way. I don't want you to do the experiment of going on a diet devoid of life energy to prove what happens. I am asking you to deduce logically what you know intuitively — lively foods make you lively. They protect life. They make you vibrant. They help the body to function normally. Having experienced this in some small part, you can understand how to maximize your knowledge of this first principle and apply it in moving toward your own ultimate diet.

A *vaidya* or expert in Ayurveda summarizes this principle of life energy as follows: "Don't eat dead or dumb foods." I have listed below what this may mean in practical terms for your diet.

Maximize Your Knowledge

Life Energy

In order to maximize your application of this principle of life energy, I suggest the following:

<u>Avoid Dead Foods</u>
Dead foods Include:

    A. Leftovers
    B. Frozen foods
    C. Canned foods
    D. Prepackaged foods
    E. Dead animal tissues

<u>Avoid Dumb Foods</u>
Dumb foods are foods that require some "doctoring" to make you think that they are good-tasting and fresh. The intelligence that gives that good, fresh taste is lost, and chemicals are added to try to imitate it. Dumb foods are foods with:

    A. Preservatives
    B. Artificial flavors
    C. Artificial coloring

Obviously, some of these recommendations require an explanation. "What is a leftover?" is a question I often hear. For the purist, any food that is not eaten immediately after it is prepared starts to lose some of its life energy. Realistically it is okay to eat food up to four to six hours later, as long as you haven't put it in the refrigerator. The best would be to eat only freshly prepared food. Any guideline like this must be taken as a goal. Know the principle — know what is best — then move in that direction.

In avoiding dead foods, the mention of "dead animal tissue" raises the fur on many. The reality of the meat-based American diet is that it is largely an experimental diet. At no time in the history of humanity have people eaten a primarily meat-based diet. (Even the "hunters and gatherers" of ancient ages did more gathering than hunting.) The results of this experiment are being reaped in terms of disease and poor health.

THE SCIENCE BEHIND THE SAGES

EFFECTS OF FOOD PROCESSING ON LIFE ENERGY

Kirlian photography has also been used to assess the effect of different processing methods on food products.

The results of natural food processing revealed strong electroluminescence (i.e., life force) in raw foods and after wok cooking and steaming. Pressure-cooking, prolonged boiling, deep-frying, barbecuing and grilling, and oven baking demonstrated increasingly diminishing electroluminescence patterns. Microwave cooking is **not** a natural technique of processing foods and, hence, should be avoided at all cost. Abundant scientific data from other fields have shown the detrimental effect of microwave cooking on the molecular structure of foods.

With regard to food storage, Kirlian photography revealed that fresh raw foods had significantly more energy. Raw foods stored in the refrigerator for four hours had the next highest. Foods subjected to Freeze-drying and freezing retained 75% and 30% of their original energy, respectively. The Kirlian-field was totally obliterated by gamma radiation.

It is predictable that if dead foods take away from ones energy and health, a diet based on dead animal tissues will be a prescription for disease. I know this is stating it harshly. The reality is that sufficient research has shown undeniably that vegetarians are healthier. This is not meant to be judgmental. In fact, if you are not a vegetarian, I don't recommend that you become one overnight. Changing too fast can cause problems. But I do encourage you to recognize that moving in the direction of a vegetarian diet is important for your health and consistent with the basic principle that lively foods convey life energy. This is not just some cultist recommendation from Ayurvedic Medicine. This theme runs through almost any ancient medical tradition. While the qualities of meats are understood and described and are even sometimes recommended for certain disease states, no tradition recommends a meat-based diet. This is particularly so if you are pursuing a spiritual path. Some evidence supporting this way of eating comes from modern science and is described below.

THE SCIENCE BEHIND THE SAGES

FYI: VEGETARIAN DIET

Vegetarians fare better than nonvegetarians in terms of a number of health measures. In addition, they are less prone to some of the most common "modern" diseases. Below is a brief summary of some of the advantages of a vegetarian diet.

Vegetarianism — Reduced Risks:

1. Hypertension
Vegetarians have repeatedly been found to have lower blood pressure than those who eat meat. The incidence of hypertension in one study was 2% in vegetarians versus 26% in adult meat-eaters. Adding meat to the diets of vegetarians raises their blood pressure. Putting hypertensive meat-eaters on a vegetarian diet results in small but significant decreases in blood pressure.

2. Coronary Artery Disease (Heart Disease)
Mortality from coronary artery disease is lower in vegetarians. A study of 25,000 Californians carried out over a 20-year period showed meat consumption was directly related to a higher incidence of fatal heart attacks in both men and women, even after other factors such as obesity were controlled for. In men 45 to 64 there were 3 times as many fatal heart attacks in meat-eaters. Vegetarians have lower total serum cholesterol, lower triglycerides, and lower levels of low-density (LDL) cholesterol.

3. Diabetes (Type II)
Diabetes as the underlying cause of death is only half as likely in vegetarians according to one study. In countries where diet is basically vegetarian, the incidence of diabetes is low. When people in these countries switch to a meat-based diet, the incidence of diabetes increases.

THE SCIENCE BEHIND THE SAGES (cont.)

4. Cancer
Cancer rates are lower for vegetarians, especially cancer of the breast and colon. Cancer of the prostate is less frequent in those whose diets are lower in fats and protein and richer in vegetables. Lung cancer incidence is less in vegetarians, even when smoking is accounted for.

5. Osteoporosis
Bone loss in vegetarian women age 65 is 18% versus 35% for meat-eaters in several studies. Cross-cultural studies also suggest an advantage for bone health for vegetarians.

6. Pesticide Toxicity
Foods of animal origin are the major source of pesticide residues in the diet. 95% to 99% of all toxic chemical residues come from meat, fish, dairy products, and eggs.

7. Obesity
Vegetarians are leaner than nonvegetarians. Their weights are closer to desirable levels, especially among vegans.

Along with some of the recipes at the end of the book, an easy method for making the transition to vegetarianism is presented. Gradual transition is key and can be quite enjoyable (and even make you feel better).

In teaching my patients, I have found several practical considerations worth mentioning. These address the mechanics of fitting fresh food, freshly prepared into the American lifestyle.

The most common misperception is that it is healthier to undertake a "raw foods" diet. Certainly, nothing could be fresher. But conveying lively energy *to* the body is not simply a matter of putting lively food *in* the body. This energy and essence must be transferred to the body. This process involves being able to break down the food.

Most people do not realize that the human body lacks the enzymes to break down cellulose — the major constituent of the surface of most vegetables and fruits. Fruits have cells that are easily broken, and the essence of the plant can often be easily absorbed. So, our orange juice can be squeezed out of the orange. Try squeezing the juice out of a piece of broccoli — it's very difficult. For that reason, the ancients recommended food be cooked so that it could be better absorbed. This does not mean cooked to death until the vegetables are limp and the nutrients destroyed. This means lightly steamed or lightly sautéed so that the essence of the food is still present.

Another reason for cooking: The raw food becomes roughage that then lines the intestinal wall, blocking the absorption of nutrients into the body. So cooking helps the process of being able to absorb the essence of the plants. It does not matter how much vitamin content is in the food you eat if you can't absorb it. The Chinese knew that raw foods could actually hinder digestion. "… excessive consumption of cold and raw foods can hinder the Spleen [digestive] function of transformation and transportation and lead to Spleen Qi deficiency. Eating at irregular times or excessive eating can also strain the Spleen capacity and lead to Spleen Qi deficiency. Eating too little or eating a protein-deficient diet can also cause Spleen deficiency." [Macciocia, Giovanni. *The Foundations of Chinese Medicine.* (Churchill Livingstone, 1989) p. 242.]

How does one get fresh food, freshly prepared and cooked? As one of my colleagues was fond of saying, "If we can put a man on the moon with 1960s technology, we ought to be able to figure out a way to have fresh food, freshly prepared in the 21st century." One of the advantages of living today is that we can rely a bit on technology, rather than on hiring a cook to follow us around all day. In the next section, I give some hints as to how this can be done.

One final misconception is in regard to grains. Grains contain the seed of life, and seeds hold onto their life energy. They are designed to do so, so that they can be planted the following year and grow a strong crop. If seeds had to be perfectly fresh to contain the life energy, they would never last until the next growing season. In this way, seeds and grains are an exception to the freshness rule.

Some methods of cooking are better than others. I will discuss microwave cooking, cooking methods, and the energy behind cooking in other chapters. To get you started with applying this first principle of life energy, I present some recipes. The first is a guaranteed way of getting that boost of energy in the morning from lively fresh fruit. The second is a general approach to "livening up" your vegetables and grains. The final recipe is actually a strategy for making the transition to a vegetarian diet in an easy and enjoyable manner.

Life energy is a key concept in Enlightened Nutrition. It is ignored in almost every diet and nutrition book. It is key to your liveliness and health. You experience this in a subtle way with things like fresh orange juice. Just like water wearing away at a rock, this subtle energy over like water wearing away at a rock, this subtle energy over time makes for health or disease. Now that you know the implications of your experience, it is time to take your experience seriously ... and to enjoy the liveliness of food.

*** Time Out: See the Stewed Apple Recipe in Appendix II***

Enjoying: Livening Up Your Food

A simple method to liven up your meals:

One of the most important principles in cooking and in Enlightened Nutrition is that taste is vitally important. It conveys the quality of the intelligence of the food and it provides much of the satisfaction that comes with eating. Therefore, learning simple ways to "spice up" your food is vitally important to diet. In fact, having all six tastes (sweet, sour, salty, bitter, astringent, pungent) in some measure is thought to be best for diet and digestion. One way to "liven up" your meals and give them fresh vibrant taste, while at the same time adding some sour and astringent taste, is to use fresh lemon or lime. Squeeze fresh lime juice on your asparagus or chard or other green vegetable for a tangy taste-enhancing treat. Or squeeze lemon on a rice dish or vegetable to give it a fresh burst of taste.

The key to changing diet is to find enjoyable new foods and new ways of preparing them. In this manner, the transition can be made easily.

Change should not be a shock. If it is too sudden it will cause stress and problems, and the change most likely will not be permanent. As you learn to liven up foods, you can start to also make the transition to a vegetarian diet. Here is what the ancients gave as a prescription for changing any habit.

THE INSIDE SCOOP

Changing Habits

Before the prescription for transition to a vegetarian diet is presented, it is important for us to note that the ancient vaidyas (expert physicians) knew that changing habits was difficult, especially when it came to eating habits. They also recognized that it can sometimes be damaging to change habits too quickly (too much of a shock to the system). For this reason, they gave the following prescription for changing habits:

Week One: Decrease undesirable habit by ¼, and increase desired habit by ¼.

Weeks Two and Three: Decrease undesirable habit by ½, and increase desired habit by ½.

Weeks Four, Five, and Six: Decrease undesirable habit by ¾, and increase desired habit by ¾.

Week Seven: Stop undesirable habit, and adopt desired habit.

The times are not set in stone. The point is to make big changes slowly, so that they can be permanent, and the mind does not rebel against them. No dietary change should be a shock to the system or involve pain or struggle.

Finally, to help with the transition to more lively and life-giving foods, the following recommendations are given to help convert to a vegetarian diet.

Enjoying: Method for Transition to Vegetarian Diet

One of the easiest ways to switch to a vegetarian diet is to explore the great ethnic foods available in this country. Vegetarian diet is not something new. Each culture is familiar with how to cook tasty meals without meat. In fact, most cultures have had a base diet that is composed of grains and legumes. For example, traditional Mexican cooking was based on corn and pinto beans. Because of this, wonderful vegetarian meals can be found among almost all ethnic foods. While I don't usually recommend restaurant food, you can get some good ideas for vegetarian meals by going to ethnic restaurants and perusing their menus. Sampling some of their foods can help to give your taste buds some wonderful surprises that will encourage you to learn to cook these foods at home.

Vegetarian diet does not mean a diet composed of vegetables. This is one of the most common misconceptions that meat-eaters have. Being a vegetarian does not mean that one is banished to eating salads for the rest of ones life. Here are some examples of vegetarian meals from the world's great ethnic cuisines:

Italian: Fettuccini Alfredo, Cheese Ravioli, Pasta Primavera
Greek: Spanikopeta, Grape Leaves
Indian: Saag Panir, Dahl, Vegetable Kofta
Mexican: Enchiladas, Vegetable Quesadilla, Burritos
Middle Eastern: Hommus, Baba Ghanush
Thai: Pad Thai, Vegetable Curry
Chinese: Fried Bean Curd with Vegetables, Vegetable Lo Mein

The Basic Strategy: Find foods you enjoy, and start to incorporate these into your diet one or two days a week. Then as you find more foods that you like, increase the number of meatless days in your week, until you find enough enjoyable foods to avoid meat altogether.

* 4 *

Food & Emotion

When consciousness and cuisine meet, life tastes good.
— Anonymous

Food and feeling go together. Despairing over "emotional eating" is a bit of a contradiction. What eating isn't emotional? Eating is one of the pleasures of physical existence — so much so that doctors observe severe depression in the elderly when they lose their sense of taste or can't eat. They observe the same thing in chemotherapy patients who lose their appetite. Food is one of the great parts of being human. Food evokes emotions and memory. Smell is one of the most sensitive triggers for memory. The smell of homemade bread or the smell of fresh-baked cookies brings forth delicious childhood memories for many people.

Eating used to be thought of as a process involving the gut or the "gastrointestinal system." We now know that the gut is lined with neuroendocrine cells — cells that produce hormone-like neuropeptides. The molecules produced by these cells have a direct effect on the brain. Just as in the expression "a gut feeling," we do actually feel with our gut. Neuropeptides produced by the gut stimulate the emotional centers in the brain. Food and emotion go hand in hand.

The understanding of this relationship between food and emotion in the ancient medical systems goes far deeper than molecular biochemistry. Just as the concept of life energy is subtle, so too are emotions. Again, it depends on awareness. The more aware you are, the more sensitive you will be to the emotional effects of foods. An experiment to understand some of the principles behind emotion and food is presented below.

Experiment #2

The Homemade Bread Experience

Required Materials:
A recipe from your mother or grandmother — it can be any baked food you remember the taste of well. Homemade bread, banana bread, or cookies will suffice.

Method:
For this experiment, it is crucial that you follow the recipe *exactly*. If the recipe calls for a brand-name ingredient, do not substitute any other brand. You must follow the recipe exactly as your mother or grandmother made it.

After the bread is out of the oven and has cooled a bit, taste it and compare what you taste to your memory. Write down your experience and contrast the difference between what you have baked and what you remember tasting in the past.

This experiment would seem to require great powers of discrimination in taste. I have consistently found that this is not the case. Almost everyone experiences something different. Again, if you are one of the few who don't experience a difference, don't get stressed out about it. (The reason you don't may become clearer as you read some other people's reactions.) Here are some of the testimonies from our patients:

"The recipe I made tasted fine, but not great, not the way I had remembered it."
— *Sam G., Accountant*

"I am a very good cook. I feel I learned this from my mother. Even before doing the experiment, though, I had known that no matter how hard I try, I can never perfectly imitate my mother's cooking."
— *Joan B., Housewife*

"At first I didn't really notice any difference between the banana bread I made and what I had remembered. They were both sweet, warm, and delicious. But with the second piece of bread I took, I did notice that it just was lacking something. It didn't have that warm feeling... It was physically warm, but it didn't warm me up... It was not as soothing is the only way I can describe it."
— *Janet C., Social Worker*

"I never feel very nourished by my own cooking. My grandmother's cooking always makes me feel nourished and loved. I just don't get that from my own cooking."
— *Laura B., Student*

Just as in the previous experiment, I pose some further questions to help you reflect on your experience and on the experiences noted above:

1) Why would it be that the exact same ingredients and the exact same method of preparation have different effects for many people?

2) Why would the emotional experience of eating one's own cooking be different from eating someone else's?

3) What is it about "homemade" food that is different from restaurant or "store bought" foods?

4) Why would someone else's cooking feel more nourishing than your own? Since you are using ingredients that are baked and eating them fresh out of the oven, you cannot conclude that the difference has to do with freshness or life energy. Some other factor must be at play. Mother's cooking just tastes different. But why?

THE INSIDE SCOOP

Food & Consciousness

Food was not thought of in terms of pure nutrition value by the ancient seers. Food is part of a living system. It is considered alive (when not old and frozen). Just like plants and animals, food is thought to have consciousness. Plants are affected by how they are handled, as are animals. One dramatic example of this was a study on cholesterol in rabbits. Researchers were feeding a group of rabbits a high-fat, atherosclerosis-producing diet. They wanted to produce atherosclerosis to research the effects of an intervention on the rabbits' coronary arteries. However, they kept having problems producing atherosclerosis in one group of rabbits. This puzzled the researchers, because the rabbits in their lab were all the same type of rabbits and all on the same diet. Yet, one group kept having normal arteries. They decided to research the problem and discovered that all the healthy rabbits were under the care of the same graduate student. They assumed the graduate student was doing something wrong in feeding the diet to the rabbits, so they decided to observe all the rabbit handlers. What they found was that all the handlers were following the dietary feeding instructions perfectly, but that the one graduate student who cared for the rabbits in question loved rabbits. When he would go to feed the rabbits he would take them out, pet them, talk to them, and play with them. The researchers then realized that the qualities of the handlers were as important as the quality of the food.

In a similar manner, the ancient seers realized that the qualities of the cook and the cook's thoughts during cooking are crucial factors in health. For that reason, many spiritual masters have been very picky about who cooks for their disciples. They insist on very spiritual cooks who have their attention on spirituality during cooking. This aspect of many retreat centers is overlooked in the U.S. when compared with the ashrams of India.

The popular book *The Secret Lives of Plants* details many of the ways in which plants are sensitive to human beings and human interactions. They are sensitive to energies, to sounds and vibrations. For example, one study showed that plants tend to grow differently when different music is played. Dr. Hari Sharma played hard rock to one set of plants and classical Indian music (*gandharva veda*) to another. The results? The plants grew away from the speakers when rock music was played. They grew toward the speakers when the gandharva music was played.

This scientific knowledge hints at the ancient knowledge of living systems. The sages knew that living things are more than containers of life energy. They are also conveyors or transmitters of mental, emotional, and spiritual energy (consciousness). Just as a molecule contains energy in the bonds between atoms, it also conveys certain qualities to the body through its structure. In the subtle world, energy can take on the vibrations that are in the environment and convey these to others.

To the ancients, it was second nature that one person's cooking would have a different quality from the next person's. They saw that the living substance took on some of the energies and vibrations of the cook. That is why no one can fully duplicate your mother's chocolate chip cookies. The cookies contain the same ingredients. Your taste buds still function. Your memory is not deceiving you. The cook is the difference. And a mother's cooking is very different because mothers love their children, and that love is conveyed through the cooking.

This knowledge leads to our second major principle of Enlightened Nutrition:

Principle #2: Food Conveys Emotion and Consciousness

Emotion is a key component of a meal. The emotion we feel coming from the food is important. This is an important part of what nourishes us. It is the emotional feeling we have after a meal that is as important as the content of the nutrients in the food. Without the feeling of satisfaction and of nurturing, a meal falls flat. We simply are not satisfied. A vague feeling of wanting more ensues.

Nature works on many levels simultaneously. The biochemical level is one part of the physical level. Food contains biochemical substances. When burned, these substances produce consistently measurable amounts of energy or calories. Food also conveys information and intelligence on emotion and spiritual levels. Admittedly, it is subtle. But subtle does not mean unimportant.

When you walk in the house of a friend, you immediately pick up a feeling. The feeling is subtle, but very palpable if you attend to it. Any real estate agent will tell you that the feeling you have walking into a home is *very* important in terms of whether that home will sell. To encourage this, some realtors recommend baking a pie in the oven before a showing, so that the house evokes memories of pleasant smells in the potential buyers.

Emotion rides on the waves of material substance. A radio amplifies a subtle energy, and it also conveys a certain vibration through that amplification. We saw in the previous chapter that food is a source of life energy. Just like the radio, the vibrational quality of that energy is altered by what the cook was "tuned into." If they were tuning into a loving feeling and excitement about creating a great-tasting dish for someone, then a wonderful feeling is conveyed in the food. If they were hurriedly trying to prepare the food, feeling frustrated about not getting paid enough by some greedy restaurant owner, that food would perhaps satisfy the palate but not the emotions. On a subtle level one will be left craving something more ... that other dessert ... an after dinner drink ... a piece of chocolate ...

Food conveys the consciousness of the cook. By consciousness, I mean the sum of the vibrations flowing through the conscious and unconscious mind of the cook, as well as the field underlying these vibrations. This is abstract because it is rarely experienced clearly, but you may have experienced this in the last exercise. Nevertheless, it is an important component of how food "works."

THE SCIENCE BEHIND THE SAGES

FOOD CONVEYS CONSCIOUSNESS

Food conveys the state of mind of the individuals who grew, harvested, and prepared the food.

Three examples demonstrating the effect of positive consciousness on the structure and taste of water are presented below. Why water? It most efficiently conducts *prana*, or life energy.

Example 1:
Individuals were asked to project loving thoughts into water. The effect of this was tested subjectively as well as objectively. The subjective test asked individuals to drink from identical cups of water. They *all* reported that the water "infused with love" tasted sweeter when compared to the "control." The objective test examined the water with nuclear magnetic resonance equipment. It revealed that the bond angle of the oxygen and hydrogen in water "infused with love" was actually changed.

Example 2:
Dr. Masuru Emoto filled bottles with water, exposed them to words, music, or prayer, and then froze them. He then photographed the resulting crystals. The structure of the crystal directly reflected the quality of source it was exposed to. The word "war" produced a fuzzy, irregular crystal. Words reflecting positive consciousness (i.e., "mother's cooking," "love," and "thanks") generated brilliant, symmetrical crystals. Similarly, crystal formation reflected the source where the water was obtained. For example, contaminated bodies of water near major cities produced irregular crystals. ["He Talks to Water" in Utne (Sept/Oct 2004, No. 125, p. 73)]

THE SCIENCE BEHIND THE SAGES (Cont.)

Example 3:
Dr. Bernard Grad, a biologist at McGill University in Montreal, used objective measures to demonstrate that water can be structured with healing intent. He reported that the absorption spectrum, surface tension, conductivity, and acidity of water can be altered by focused thought (intent). The scientific explanation is as follows: The hydrogen bond angles of the structured water molecule widen, thereby weakening the normal attraction of water molecules to one another. This,s in turn, decreases the surface tension and increases the solubility of the structured water. An altered spectrum-absorption pattern is recorded. [In Laskow, Healing with Love, p. 35; citing Gerber, Vibrational Medicine, p. 295]

The effect of consciousness on plant form:

Dr. Grad experimented on the effect of positively and negatively structured water and its effects on the growth of plants. Individuals were asked to simply hold water containers in their hands, thereby structuring water. Water was positively structured by an individual reputed to have a "green thumb." Water was negatively structured by a severely depressed mental patient. Plants were regularly treated with either the positively (green thumb) or negatively (depressed patient) structured water or with plain water. The results: Everything else being equal, the plants that received the green thumb's structured water grew faster than those that received plain water. Plants that received the depressed patient's structured water grew more slowly than the plants that received plain water. [In Laskow, Healing with Love, p. 35; citing Gerber, Vibrational Medicine, p. 295]

Other examples of this principle of living things acting as carriers for vibrations come from homeopathy. In this healing art, a plant or mineral extract is placed in water but then diluted so many times that not a single molecule of the original substance is left. The water is pure from a chemical view. From the homeopathic view, however, it has taken on the vibrations of the substance and acts as a carrier. Randomized clinical trials have shown that these "inert" waters have effects far beyond those of placebo. Water is not the only medium for conveying vibrations. Food is a powerful medium for conveying the consciousness of the cook.

What is the emotion and intention of food prepared at McDonald's, Wendy's, or other fast-food establishments? What is the consciousness and spiritual development of the average cook at a fast-food restaurant? What is his or her intention? What is the intention of the owner? Even meals produced at a fancy restaurant have different vibrations from those of someone who loves you. The intention of most restaurant owners is to make money. This is "the American way." That intention though is something that is communicated to all who eat there. That is why a home-cooked meal is different from restaurant food.

Much of the craving for sugar and sweetness is because the food one eats lacks this subtle quality of nourishment and nurturance. Emotional eating ensues not only when one is upset, but also when food is lacking in emotional value. Certainly, when one is stressed, the craving to feel calmer and nourished is greater. But when food is devoid of nurturing vibrations, it won't nourish one on an emotional level. The stomach will be full, but the heart will be empty. This situation can only further contribute to emotional eating. The emotions will not be satisfied, and the craving for more sweet, more salt, more interesting flavors will become exaggerated.

The future will see the role of cook placed on a very high level next to that of doctor or healer. The cook will know what is needed to balance and promote health. Cooking will be undertaken with a reverence for life that communicates the highest love and spirituality to those who partake of the food. Cooks will be honored, respected, and well-paid.

I started the chapter by stating that all eating is emotional eating. This was not to make light of the fact that many people under stress eat in ways that are unhealthy. Emotional eating occurs when stress is not attended to properly. Meditation helps to deal with the stress in many ways because relaxation is one of its by-products. This fact is so well-known that many mistake meditation for relaxation techniques. In fact, meditation is to develop awareness. Meditation expands one's awareness and sensitivity to the subtle aspects of existence, including the food we eat.

One solution to emotional eating is to deal with stress through meditation practice. Another is to develop the habit of eating foods that are cooked with positive emotion. That means eating foods cooked by someone loving and spiritual. If you can find that at a nearby restaurant—great. Most likely, though, you'll need to start at home to find this rare quality.

Maximize Your Knowledge

Optimal Eating

1. Eat in a settled environment.

2. Eat in an emotionally uplifting environment.

3. Try sharing cooking with a friend or neighbor, rather than going out to restaurants.

4. Do not cook or eat when upset (food will not digest properly). Cooking with uplifting emotion and caring feeling makes a difference.

5. Eat slowly enough to *experience* food — you can't be emotionally nourished if you don't experience the food, so do not rush your meals.

6. No TV while eating.

7. No reading while eating.

8. Sit for a minimum of five minutes after meals, although ten minutes is preferred.

Listed below are several recipes that convey caring. They require preparation and that preparation can convey one's feelings of love and nurturance to anyone who eats the food.

Our first two principles have been abstract, but your experience makes them concrete. Attending to your experience and valuing it can make all the difference in how you live and eat. Good health, after all, is abstract.

When you have it, though, you feel it and know it. Embracing these abstract principles will make all the difference in how you feel, and emotion is central to life and to food.

Enjoying: Foods That Convey Caring

Date Shake

INGREDIENTS:
- 4-5 whole dates (Medjool variety or similar is best)
- 1 cup whole organic milk
- 2 pinches cinnamon powder

INSTRUCTIONS:
1. Boil milk until it foams once. Turn off heat. Cool until drinkable.
2. Put milk, cinnamon, and dates in a blender.
3. Blend until dates are ground fine.
4. Serve warm in winter, room temp or slightly cool (not cold) in summer or if strong pitta imbalance (heat or inflammation in the body).

Date Raisin Chutney

INGREDIENTS:
- 1 ½ tsp fennel seeds
- 1 ½ tsp cumin seeds
- 3 tsp ground coriander
- 1 ½ cups raisins
- ¾ cup dates, (pitted, chopped)
- ½ cup orange juice
- 3 Tbsp fresh ginger root (minced)
- 3/8 tsp salt
- 4 ½ Tbsp fresh cilantro

INSTRUCTIONS:
Combine all ingredients in a food processor, and pulse until coarsely ground.

* 5 *

Re-creating the Body

By eating I become sick. By digesting I become healthy.
— Arabian saying

Look in the mirror. That person you see looks so familiar. That person was not there a year ago. Every single molecule you observe was not there a year ago. In a marvelous display of intelligence, each molecule in your face has been deftly replaced without you knowing it. You have the illusion of sameness. Just as if we gradually replaced every brick in your house silently at night, you might not recognize that you have a new house at the end of the year. The structure is the same. The layout is the same. But the house would be totally new. Imagine this happening every year. That is what happens not only with your face, but, your entire body.

Scientists have discovered a way to label carbon atoms, so that they can gauge the turnover of cells in the body. The lining of the stomach is thought to turn over every five days. This means you have a new lining to the stomach every week. The liver also has this capacity for regeneration. When undergoing surgery to remove a lobe of the liver, it is not uncommon for it to grow back in less than six months. Even that most permanent-appearing part of us, our skeleton, is not static. It is in a very dynamic state, constantly growing new bone and destroying old bone.

The entire body (or at least 98% of it) is transformed and replaced each year. Even those cells that are thought to be permanent, such as nerve cells, are replaced. Because these cells don't regenerate, the replacement process is not so obvious. But it occurs. Just like replacing the bricks in your house, the molecules that make up the components of the nerve cell are replaced over the period of a year's time.

Understanding the transformations that take place is *not* the forte of modern medicine. In contrast, we will see that ancient medical systems had detailed knowledge of the how the body's tissues are created and how food is transformed into structure. The body is a process. Understanding that process is not always in our awareness. I use the following experiment to give more insight and experience with the permeability of the body and its processes.

WARNING

This experiment is not for the faint of heart. You really have to love garlic to enjoy this experiment. Garlic taken this way can irritate the stomach, so feel free to just skip to the section on others' experiences and live vicariously. Another experiment is offered that you can substitute that does not require so much courage.

Experiment #3
The Garlic Experience

Materials Required:
1 very fresh clove of garlic.

Method:
Peel the clove and cut it into 4 quarters.
Place the garlic in your mouth and chew for 10 seconds.
Do not swallow any garlic.
Spit out the garlic.
Rinse your mouth with water.
Brush your teeth with toothpaste and rinse liberally.

Evaluation:
Write down your experience. Pay particular attention to the smell on your breath.

Here is an alternative experiment:

Experiment #3a
The Peppermint Experience

Materials Required:
1 small bottle of peppermint essential oil

Method:
Put 3-4 drops in 1 tablespoon sesame oil. Hold your nose and have someone massage the oil into your feet for five to 10 minutes.

Evaluation:
Write down your experience. Pay particular attention to the taste in your mouth.

I admit the garlic experience is least pleasant of the experiments we have tried. On the scale of things, however, it is not horrendous — just a bit smelly. Here are the reactions of some of our bolder patients:

"I knew from my past experience with garlic it wouldn't help to brush my teeth. Somehow the smell gets into you and doesn't go away."
— David W.

"My breath still reeked of garlic even though I brushed my teeth twice! I couldn't lose the smell. It was curious. I didn't even eat any. I made sure of that. But the smell somehow just got in me."
— Tonia S.

"I had read somewhere that you can smell garlic on your toes the minute you bite into a clove of garlic. I had trouble verifying that because … well, I could't get anyone to smell my feet at first, and my breath was so full of garlic smell I couldn't discern if it was coming from my mouth or my feet. Later I found a very generous volunteer who verified that indeed my feet did smell of garlic."
— Mike G.

"My experience was one of the garlic seeming to act like I had eaten it. It was entering into my body without me even eating it. It seemed to be becoming part of me even though I spit it out."
— Danielle A.

"I am not a big fan of garlic. It sort of burned in my mouth. The smell seemed to linger for hours on my breath. It was curious how penetrating garlic must be to become a part of me so fast."
— Tom M.

Many people are surprised that you don't have to actually eat the garlic for the smell to become a part of your body. How does that take place? Why would just chewing on a clove of garlic affect even the sweat on someone's feet (or the taste in the mouth when one massages in peppermint oil)?

The experiments I have presented thus far have asked you to think in terms of awareness and feeling. It has been a very intuitive orientation. Here I am asking you to analyze your experience in more concrete terms. What is happening in the body to create this experience of persistent smell? I will give you a clue: It has to do with the fact that in the mouth and under the tongue are some very exposed blood vessels.

Garlic is very penetrating in its smell. But it is not just that you can't clean it off your teeth like a very sticky glue; it is because it penetrates into the body. It does this by entering the bloodstream. The blood vessels in the mouth are a route for medicines and vitamins, as well as for pungent smelling herbs. The garlic juice you created by chewing up the garlic clove entered through the blood vessels under the tongue and elsewhere in the mouth directly into the body. The blood is carried to the tissues of the body. It nourishes the muscles and fat tissues. It gets into the lymphatics. It is processed in each part of the body. The blood that nourishes the skin supplies the various layers of the skin and eventually gets processed in the sweat glands. Eventually this smell appears in the sweat.

Blood nourishes each of the tissues of the body. One tissue affects the next tissue. How this takes place was one of the fortes of the ancient physicians.

This experience of the immediate affect of a food on the body, its blood, and its tissues leads to our next principle:

Principle #3: Food Immediately Starts Re-creating the Body

Garlic has potent and impressive qualities. It is an antibiotic. It has antiviral properties. It alters fat metabolism. It has a heating and drying effect. And it has spiritual properties as well. All of these effects and more are carried to all of the cells of the body. Anyone who has eaten a substantial amount of garlic in one sitting knows that one gets thirsty because of its drying effect. In just this way, all food immediately carries its properties to the entire body. Food alters the processes of transformation and eventually alters how the tissues of the body are formed. The seers could perceive this process and described it in detail.

The Western mind thinks in terms of parts and pieces. It gravitates toward things rather than processes. When it breaks down complex processes into things, it often loses the connections between them. Imagine two children looking through a fine slit in the wall. A cat walks by. First, they see a head. Then they see a tail. After every head comes a tail. They conclude that a head causes the tail to appear. This is because they don't see the head and tail as part of a single "cat" process.

In that manner, the actual tissue layers perceived by the ancients are not what is important. It is not what I can name and see, but it is the process of transformation that is important. If you can't transform what you eat properly into well-formed tissues, you have the stage set for disease. Another word for transforming food is digestion. What I mean by this is far beyond burning calories. Digestion is the process through which we re-create the body. Its importance is unsurpassed.

On a trip to China to visit a college of natural medicine, I was taken by surprise by a comment about the expensive urine in the United States. It seemed an odd comment and at first sounded like a mistranslation. The importance of transformation in order to utilize food properly brings home the point. Many Americans consume very expensive vitamins and supplements. Because digestion is poor, these are never absorbed and incorporated into the body. The supplements are simply excreted in the urine. It is the process of transformation and absorption that is important, not the number of milligrams of a substance you pop in your mouth.

How does one tissue transform and nourish the next? The Ayurvedic seers taught that each tissue has a "fire of transformation" or its own digestive process. These "fires" of digestion allow one tissue to nourish and transform into the next tissue. From our fragmented and "thing-oriented" way of thinking, this sounds fanciful. How does fat "become" bone? What does bone marrow have to do with the nervous system? Analyzing the tissues from the knowledge of Western science can help to answer these questions.

Plasma to Blood Cells

Blood cells are bathed in plasma. Digested food is absorbed into the blood stream and is carried in plasma and thus nourishes and supports blood cells.

Blood Cells to Muscle Tissue

Blood cells affect the next tissue layer, the muscle tissue (*mamsa*). Red blood cells carry oxygen to the muscle tissue for aerobic metabolism. White blood cells help to carry off debris from dying cells and supply many of the immune functions that protect the body from bacteria and viruses.

Muscle Tissue to Fat Tissue

What happens when old football players retire? What happens when you stop working out? Often weight remains stable, but the muscle "turns to fat." This transformation comes about because of an increased nourishment of the fatty tissue layer when the previous layer (muscle tissue) no longer requires so many nutrients.

Fat Tissue to Bone

This is one of the hardest for people to conceptualize. Remember this is a process, not a "thing." The key to understanding this is to realize that the cholesterol molecule is the biochemical "backbone" or building block for many of the major hormones in the body. In fact, 25% of estrogen production in women comes not from the ovaries, rather from fat stores. Many hormonal functions are ascribed to this "fatty tissue layer" in classical Ayurvedic teachings. Estrogen is very nourishing to bone. It causes bone growth. That was formerly one of the major reasons for promoting hormone replacement therapy in women. Several other tissue layers are described in the classics of Ayurveda and are similarly recognized in Tibetan Medicine and as well as in Chinese and Japanese Medicine. Even with our limited knowledge of the body, modern science has started to make connections that verify the seers' knowledge of the tissues of the body. What does this knowledge emphasize? It recognizes the importance of digestion at each tissue layer. If digestion is not adequate, the body is not nourished even when the best and purest foods are taken. Digestion is of paramount importance in the ancient systems of medicine. Without it, the body cannot properly re-create itself. Our experiment with garlic demonstrated how quickly food is transformed and influences the tissues of the body. It also shows that when we cannot fully break down and transform a substance, it can show up in our sweat, our breath, and our skin, and it can create offensive smells.

Digestion is paramount to health. Proper formation of the tissues cannot take place without it. Digestion and transformation of each of the tissues into the next layer is crucial for health and longevity. Diet ultimately involves the food eaten, the eater's ability to digest, and the process of transformation. Enlightened Nutrition involves the ultimate processing of what is taken in. Without that, nothing we eat can nourish us.

The good news: Digestion can be improved. The process by which we transform food into healthy tissue can be enhanced. We generally ignore this aspect in modern nutrition. We focus on calories and nutrients and don't recognize that each of the steps in the process of re-creating the body can be aided and optimized. The "fires of digestion" responsible for the nourishment of each tissue layer can be improved. The ancient seers cognized general ways to improve digestion, as well as specific formulas that target each "fire." From the perspective of Chinese Medicine it is important to "protect the Spleen Qi." This means one should take steps to assure its ability to function is not damaged. It is seen as the major source of energy and nourishment after birth.

Maximize Your Knowledge

Optimizing Digestion

In order to gain the most from this principle of re-creating the body through proper digestion, it is advised that you do the following:

Optimize Digestive Strength:
- Eat when you are hungry.
- Don't eat when you aren't hungry.
- Eat to only 75% full.
- Don't eat until the previous meal is digested (3 - 6 hours).
- Avoid large amounts of liquid before, after, or during meals.
- Make lunch the large meal of the day.
- Avoid ice-cold food and beverages.
- Chew well.
- Avoid large quantities of raw and uncooked food.
- Do not eat when you are upset.
- Do not eat too quickly or too slowly.

Optimize the Digestive Environment:
- Eat in a settled, quiet atmosphere with a settled mind.
- Do not work, read, or watch TV while eating.
- Always sit to eat.
- Eat at approximately the same times each day.
- Take a few minutes to sit quietly after a meal before returning to activity.
- Don't eat right before bed.
- Take food that is pleasant to both sight and palate.
- Take food that is prepared by a happy, settled cook.

If you look at the suggestions in the above section optimizing digestion, you will note that *how* you eat is as important as *what* you eat. The seers understood this and they emphasized this. But this was in addition to the amazingly potent herbal formulas they prescribed for improving digestion. Too often, we become "pill-oriented." Health is not in a pill, whether it is an herb pill or a drug pill. Herbs and drugs can help, but only when we are in tune with our true nature.

The Chinese saw the etiology of weakness in the ability to digest as having many etiologies. How you eat and how you live can influence the strength of digestion or the "Qi of the Spleen": "Excessive thinking or mental strain over a long period of time can cause Spleen Qi deficiency. This is common in students or business people who spend long periods of time every day in mental work. This is particularly harmful if one goes back to work straight after a hurried lunch, or even worse, conducts business over lunch." [Macciocia, Giovanni. *The Foundations of Chinese Medicine.* (New York: Churchill Livingstone, 1989) p. 243.]

Before I discuss some recipes for digestion, I would like to address some of the above recommendations. Invariably, I have seen that when people are given a long set of guidelines, they will tend to treat them as rules. Now we all react differently to rules … and that is the point. Some people will tend to drive themselves nuts following each exactly and then feel guilty if they stray. Some find them overwhelming and conclude this approach is not for them. Some drive their relatives nuts with their newfound knowledge. Some try the rules for a while and then rebel.

The emphasis in this book is self-awareness. I am encouraging subjective knowledge. I am trying to have you refer to your experience and to yourself. These guidelines represent things to try. Your experience in trying them will serve as a guide. As you pay attention to how you feel, you will begin to understand why the seers recommended these ways to help digestion. You will know which are important for your particular physical makeup.

Even so, I often am asked to prioritize these by my students and patients. Given this, let me offer a brief discussion of the most important points regarding digestion.

1. Eat when you are hungry.

And don't eat when you are not hungry. This is probably the most important point in protecting digestion and assimilating food. When you are hungry, the body is ready to process food. The production of digestive enzymes is maximal. The intensity of stomach acidity is greater. The food can be moved through the gut most easily. When you are hungry and ignore the urge to eat, the body starts to go into fasting mode and begins to digest fat stores. This actually suppresses hunger. It weakens the intensity of digestion over time. The seers taught that digestion was like a fire. If you don't put any fuel on it, it goes out. If you put just a little fuel on it, it cannot burn brightly.

One important point: You must learn to distinguish between the sensation of hunger and the desire to have something that would "entertain" the palate. The mind would enjoy some chocolate or some ice cream, but is the gut empty? Is the stomach growling and hungry?

Hunger comes from the gut, not from the brain. Entertainment comes from the brain. Cravings for this taste or that taste usually represent some imbalance that is forcing the mind to think of food. This is different from being hungry.

Not eating when you aren't hungry is just as important. The body handles the processing of food in a stepwise fashion. If one is not hungry, it means either one of the steps is incomplete or the body is doing some "internal housekeeping" before it can digest another meal. When you are not hungry, the stomach does not have strong acid to break down food. The amount of digestive enzymes available is less. The body cannot break food down properly.

Imagine a conveyor belt at a large manufacturing company. Each person on the assembly line has responsibility for putting one part onto the machine. Each can only put the right part on at the right time. Say you are in the middle of assembling a car. Imagine what happens on the assembly line when someone plunks down a new chassis right in the middle of a half-assembled car. The workers either stop working on the car they have half assembled, or they start working on the new chassis. In the best case, they get one of the two done. In the worst case, both are ruined. Digestion is much more complex than this, but it takes place in a similar stepwise fashion. If you are not done digesting the previous meal (if you have no hunger), then you are dumping a new chassis on top of a half-assembled car. Not only will the food get wasted, the body will get overwhelmed with what to do with the waste.

This waste actually creates problems for the body. (I'll talk more about that in the next chapter.) When this waste builds up sufficiently, you can lose appetite altogether. The body will then digest some of the built-up waste. This is the principle behind fasting. Unfortunately, many people will have disturbing symptoms as the body starts to clean house. They get a headache, they get light-headed, or they feel they can't function. Many people eat to prevent these things from happening. The worst of this is when people eat every couple of hours to prevent becoming "hypoglycemic." They start to experience some of the symptoms of internal housecleaning and stop the process out of fear. This further damages digestion and assures they will never get the body back to a state of balance.

This guideline sounds so simple. For many, it is the hardest to apply. For everyone, it is key.

2. Try to make lunch the main meal of the day.

This is difficult in our culture. Try it for a week. You can do almost anything for a week. Most likely, you'll notice a difference. How can you do this without hiring a personal chef? The easy answer is to just eat more at lunch and less at dinner. If you are used to taking a sandwich for lunch, take two sandwiches. If you are used to eating a plateful of food at night, take just half a plateful. Why? Digestion goes in cycles along with our biorhythms. It is most effective at certain times of day. Noontime is when the body's digestion is strongest. It is optimal and is able to handle large meals.

Nighttime is not so good for digestion. The closer to bedtime we eat, the less likely the body will be able to fully process food. This results in many problems. One of the most common is acid reflux or gastroesophageal reflux disease (GERD). In this condition, food comes back up from the stomach into the esophagus. The acid from the stomach can burn the esophagus and can even come so high up that it burns and irritates the throat. Billions of dollars are spent each year on medication for this condition. Many cases could be avoided if people just made this one simple change — taking the large meal of the day at noon.

In the evening when digestion is weak, taking a large meal will lead to the accumulation of toxins in the body. This recommendation requires no herbs or any money whatsoever. It can give one new energy. It can improve sleep. It can prevent heartburn. Even some weight gain can be prevented by taking meals at a time when the calories can be burned, rather than at night when they are more readily stored.

How does one have a hot meal at lunch in the middle of the day? One simple way to accommodate a busy work schedule is to use modern conveniences like a crockpot, rice maker, or thermos. On the following page is a favorite recipe for a hot and nourishing lunch.

Enjoying: Thermos Lunch

¼ cup	red lentils
¼ cup	basmati rice
1-1 ½ cup	fresh zucchini and/or yellow squash, (you can add small amounts of asparagus or carrots)
1 tsp	ghee or olive oil
2 cups	water
¼ tsp	fennel seeds
¼ tsp	cumin seeds
¼ tsp	ground coriander
¼ tsp	turmeric
2 pinches	salt

- Rinse the lentils and rice and put in water and bring to a boil.
- Briefly (20 seconds) sauté the spices in ghee or olive oil.
- Add the chopped vegetables and sauté for 1 minute.
- Add the vegetables and spices to the lentils and rice and simmer for 5 minutes.
- While still boiling, pour the mixture into a 1-quart thermos.
- Close the thermos quickly and leave closed for about four hours.

Notes

- You may need to experiment with cooking times depending on your thermos' ability to retain heat.

- Heavier vegetables like carrots and beets need one to two more minutes of cooking with the rice and beans.

- You can substitute yellow moong beans for red lentils.

- Do not overheat ghee when frying spices—it should not be smoking hot. Begin with whole spices and fry only to light brown or when seeds start to pop, then add ground spices for a few seconds only.

Many traditional cultures eat the main meal at noontime. They know what the ancients knew — the digestive fire is greatest at lunchtime. Our slavish work schedules have disrupted this important aspect of family life and health.

3. Eat with awareness.

This is the most important point of all. The only way the body can communicate effectively with you is through sensation and desire. If you have no idea what the body is sensing and what it is craving, you cannot hope to act in tune with its needs. If you are watching TV or reading while you eat you cannot be attending to the sensations in your body. If you are distracted by an argument or a political debate over dinner, you cannot feel the impact of that last morsel you just placed in your mouth. Awareness is key to the feeling of satisfaction. Some people will eat an entire meal and will have tasted none of it. They have no experience of having eaten. Is it any wonder that they still feel hungry after filling the stomach?

In almost every culture in the world, it is tradition to give thanks to Nature or to God or to a Higher Power for providing all that goes into making and bringing food to the table. This pause to give thanks allows awareness to be brought back to oneself and sets the stage for eating consciously. Pausing after the meal also aids digestion and the feeling of satisfaction that comes from eating. After a large meal, sitting for a minimum of 10 minutes before engaging in physical or mental work is recommended. Working alters the physiological function of the body and takes important resources away from the gut into other areas of the body. Pausing also aids awareness.

Even when we do our best to follow these guides, it is not always possible to avoid hampering digestion in some fashion. Fortunately, the ancients cognized a way to benefit each aspect of digestion and transformation. While some of these are herbal formulas, herbs are not the only mechanism for enlivening digestion. Spices and food mixtures (chutneys) can be valuable also. Spices aid in the transformation processes. They also make food lively and interesting. Spices truly are "the spice of life" because these zesty little items help to add life to food. They help in getting the life out of food. They aid in transforming food into sustenance.

Chutneys are the real appetizers in the food world. Appetizers were not meant to be something you fill up on before the meal starts. They were originally designed to enhance appetite. Chutneys do just that. Two chutney recipes are presented for you to try. The first is mild and suitable for almost everyone. The other is very spicy and should not be taken by those with sensitive stomachs.

*** Time Out: See the Pineapple Chutney Recipe in Appendix II***

*** Time Out: See the Ginger Chutney Recipe in Appendix II***

These chutneys work subtly over a period of several weeks to tone up digestion and assure transformations are proper. The pineapple chutney recipe is a formula that is also good for those people with sensitive stomachs who can't handle the hot and spicy nature of the ginger chutney. Both recipes aid digestion and prevent gas and toxin buildup.

Food immediately affects the body and its processes of transformation and re-creation. These methods for influencing the re-creation of the body, for improving digestion and the quality of the tissues have long been kept secret. We are living at a great time when long-hidden secret knowledge is becoming readily available to everyone. We know intuitively how quickly foods can affect us. With further openness to experimentation, we can learn how the body is affected by food in the long term. Key to this knowledge is understanding digestion and how the body re-creates each tissue layer. What is also key is understanding what happens when this process is less than perfect. That is the subject of our next chapter.

* 6 *

Blocks To Health

If we eat wrongly, no doctor can cure us.
If we eat rightly, no doctor is needed.
— Rocine

Sara M. has been to nine different doctors. Seven of them have been specialists. She has been struggling with chronic fatigue, day in and day out. She has had more than $4,000 worth of tests. She has been advised to see a psychiatrist about her fatigue by seven of her nine doctors. The other two doctors were psychiatrists. She has taken 12 different medications to solve her problem. She has continued to work in spite of the fatigue. She has been told that she is having fatigue because she is depressed. She counters that she was not depressed when the fatigue started. She has become depressed because it seems no one can help her, and she is worried about losing her job.

She is in her mid-30's and has had a very successful marketing career. She has only recently started going to doctors. Although she has heard of Ayurvedic Medicine in the past, she has never read anything about it. She states that she is open to trying anything to get past this problem. She has already tried megadoses of vitamins and "immune enhancing" herbs. The last place she thought to look was at her digestion. She thinks she eats a good diet with lots of salads and has been on a high-protein diet to lose weight.

She is not alone. Chronic fatigue affects millions in the U.S. She is one of the more fortunate ones, because she is able to talk directly with an Ayurvedic physician who understands her situation more deeply than her other doctors. She is also fortunate in that she is open to learning about how her body functions and how digestion is crucial to so many processes in the body.

She has gained some weight recently because she has been too tired to exercise. Her physicians have already ruled out the most common causes of fatigue. She is not anemic and does not have thyroid disease. She sleeps more than she wants to but has been trying to get to bed earlier so that she gets at least eight hours of sleep a night.

When her Ayurvedic physician takes her pulse, it is clear what the problem is. She has developed blockages in the flow of energy in the body. The level of toxins from poor digestion is very high. Her diet and lifestyle, combined with her weak digestion, have caused her to form blockages that keep her from getting any energy. She is put on a toxin-reducing diet and is given herbs for digestion. Two months later she is feeling full of energy and wonders why all doctors don't know about this approach to medicine.

The toxins formed from poor digestion represent a major block to health. When digestion is not complete, toxins are formed. These toxins are called *ama* in the Ayurvedic system. In Chinese Medicine these toxins create *phlegm,* which causes *dampness* or *damp heat* as the body tries to deal with the undigested material and the toxins that block the channels. The body must then do something with these toxins, and that process takes energy.

This next experiment gives you some firsthand knowledge of monitoring for *ama* in the body. It gives you a graphic experience of what happens with digestion. Like all of the exercises in this book, not every individual will have the same experience. Most people, though, will have a deeper understanding of how digestion works after trying it. If you are lactose sensitive, you may want to sit this one out.

Experiment #4

The Milkshake Experience

This experiment is not for those who have trouble with milk products. It is a "one time" experiment, in that I do not recommend that you do this often. The reason for this will become apparent by the end of the exercise. You are to observe some of the longer-term effects of taking a milkshake in the evening.

Required Materials:
¾ cup milk
½ cup ice cream
½ tsp vanilla flavoring

Method:
1) Mix all of the ingredients in a blender for one minute.
2) Before drinking, observe your tongue in a mirror — note the amount of coating on the tongue, whether you can scrape it off with a toothbrush, what color the coating is, and whether the coating is uniform.
3) Write down your observations.
4) Drink the milkshake one hour before bedtime (the timing is important).
5) The following morning before you have done anything else, observe your tongue again and note any differences.
6) Write down your morning observations.

Here are some questions to ponder:

1) What organ system in the body does the tongue belong to?

2) Certainly if you eat something, some of the food can immediately stain the surface of the tongue, but this goes away in an hour or two. What would explain surface changes seven or nine hours later?

3) Why would one area of the tongue be more affected than the other?

4) From observing the tongue, what would appear to be the effect of taking a cold milkshake on the digestive process?

THE INSIDE SCOOP

Diagnosing Imbalance

The human body is one of the most fascinating and complex systems in all of creation. It truly is a system. Each part affects the whole. The condition of the whole affects each part. For example, the quality of skin reflects the health of the entire body. Some experts in Ayurvedic Medicine can diagnose imbalances by one look at the skin. Some can diagnose imbalances just listening to the voice.

The tongue, just like any part of the body, reflects the health and balance of the whole body. Its location in the mouth gives one the clue that it is part of the digestive tract. This is fundamental to Traditional Chinese Medicine — it is said that the tongue is the one internal organ that can be easily observed. It reflects the conditions of the other organs.

This principle of wholeness, of the parts reflecting the status of the whole, makes diagnosing imbalances far less invasive than our modern medical methods.

Before I present further discussion of this experience, here are the observations of some of our patients:

"I would describe my tongue as having grown fur overnight. It even felt furry."
— Rebecca H., Nurse

"I only noticed a little difference between before and after. I saw a white coating on the back of my tongue before I had the milkshake.

The next day I saw some increase in the amount of coating. That's all."
— Edward F., Mechanical Engineer

"I usually don't have any coating at all on the tongue. The morning after taking the shake, there was a thin white coating over the entire surface of the tongue. Some of it scraped off with a toothbrush, but some of it didn't."
— Sherry F., Homemaker

"I noticed a thick off-white coloring in the middle of the tongue on the morning after taking the milkshake. The day before the coating had been a dirty white, almost yellow, but not anywhere near as thick."
— Ted N., Mechanic

"I noticed a bunch of blotches of white slime and some thick whitish gunk on the back of my throat. I awoke feeling stiff and sleepy. It was harder than usual to get moving. I noticed a heavy feeling, like everything inside my body had almost come to a standstill. I never realized that there could be any connection between how I feel in the morning and what I ate the night before."
— Julie H., Student

The previous chapter outlined the importance of digestion and making the proper transformation from one tissue layer to the next. The tongue reflects one aspect of this digestive process. What caused that coating? If the body had processed all of the milkshake, there would have been no residual. This residual on the tongue reflects residual elsewhere. Just as the ancient seers noted, to observe the tongue is to look into the body and watch how it is functioning. The residual you see on the tongue the morning after is that which the body could not fully process. It could not digest it, and toxins are the result. One way of monitoring levels of this type of toxin is by observing the coating on the tongue. If you can't scrape off the coating, toxins are forming that may get deeper into the tissues of the body.

Just as our patient Julie H. observed, there *is* a relationship between the food you consume the day before and how you feel the next day. Actually, the effects of what you eat today are felt long into the future. The full process of transformation of food into the last stage of tissue generally takes a minimum of 28 days.

What if you can't process the food? This feeling of heaviness and fatigue is the effect of digestive toxins on the body. It makes the joints stiff and the mind dull. It takes on a life of its own and creates the breeding ground for disease. Overwhelming the body with cold, sweet, and rich things is one way to be sure to create toxins. That is the reason I said you shouldn't do this experiment very often. This brings us to our next fundamental principle.

Principle #4: When digestion is incomplete, toxins are formed that block metabolism.

The first transformation is from the digestive system to the bloodstream. Obviously, you observed and experienced that some of the milkshake didn't get transformed into blood. It appeared on the tongue as *ama* or *phlegm* (in the Chinese system of medicine). This *ama* will hinder the next meal from being absorbed and digested. It is described in classic Ayurvedic literature as a thick, sticky substance. Being sticky, it will adhere to the walls of the intestines. Obviously, this will block the proper digestion and assimilation of food.

This is not purely an Ayurvedic concept. It is a concept that is present in many other ancient systems of medicine. As mentioned previously, digestion is thought to be a function of the "spleen" in Traditional Chinese Medicine. This word is probably a mistranslation for that organ that is in that area of the body and is responsible for digestion. Probably "pancreas" is more accurate, anatomically. (The Chinese didn't do dissection so did not have the same terminology as those translating the classical texts.) In the ancient medical text "Classic of Difficulties," the spleen is described: "The spleen weighs 2 pounds and 3 ounces, it is 3 inches wide, 5 inches long and has 1/2 pound of fatty tissues surrounding it." [Macciocia, Giovanni. *The Foundations of Chinese Medicine.* (New York: Churchill Livingstone, 1989) p. 92.] Obviously, the only organ in that area of the body that fits this description is the pancreas. Many naturopaths use pancreatic enzymes to aid digestion. When digestion is weak, the spleen is said to be malfunctioning. Spleen qi deficiency is weakness of the energy of the spleen or the function of digestion. When this weakness is present, "dampness" is created. This dampness creates the same sticky thick substance in the intestines (*phlegm*) and interferes with absorption. This is the same concept as that of *ama* in Ayurvedic Medicine.

THE INSIDE SCOOP

Ama

The ancient Ayurvedic seers described ama *in great detail. They realized that it can affect the entire body and mind in different ways. The ancient Chinese also talk of* phlegm *clouding the mind. Here are some of the understandings that give a clearer definition of digestive toxins:*

Digestive Toxins:

1) The consequence of poor digestion of food OR experience.

2) Toxins that build up in the body and prevent our connecting with the body's underlying intelligence.

3) Blockages — whether in our arteries, our eyesight, our joints or our ability to experience love and happiness.

4) Improperly digested food — any toxin or waste not utilizable by the body as food.

5) Excess of any by-products of metabolism that build up in our bodies: uric acid (causes gout), components of bile (forms gallstones), etc.

6) The products of maldigestion that block the channels or shrotas.

Ama has its impact not only on the digestive system. It can eventually get lodged in the channels of the body. In the big channels, it gives rise to atherosclerosis. In the subtle channels, it gives rise to blockages in energy flow. This makes for aches and pains in the absence of a well-defined "structural disease." It also makes for fatigue and stiffness. Ultimately, it forms the breeding ground for later disease and dysfunction.

Blockages in the flow of energy is what people who do "body work" or "energy work" focus on. It is also what acupuncture concentrates on. These methods increase the flow through the channels. Sometimes this increased flow will eliminate the blockage. Sometimes increasing the flow only temporarily helps. Like increasing the pressure in a water hose to increase the flow, increasing energy does not always guarantee the blockage is removed. That is why the problem returns after the treatments are stopped. Eliminating the blockages is what is required.

How is this done? The science of purification is itself an entire discipline. Some doctors specialize in this knowledge (*panchakarma*), just as some specialize in cardiology or dermatology. This branch of knowledge gives methods for quickly purifying toxins from the system and restoring youthfulness. Its complex nature makes it beyond the scope of this book. A slower method of detoxifying does exist — a purification diet. This must be followed for one to three weeks. More information about this will be included later in the chapter.

Unfortunately, Western medicine has no concept of purification. For some reason we understand that a car needs to have an oil change to keep working properly, yet we do not apply that notion to our bodies. For the body to function day after day, year after year, without any purification is a lot to ask. Purification diets are a special application of Enlightened Nutrition. They use the principles of Enlightened Nutrition to effect important health changes. But they are not for everyone. Purification takes energy, and taking a purifying diet when you are weak will only create more problems. It is like putting even less water through that clogged hose. Maybe you will eventually dissolve the clog … but maybe not. And if you don't, then the flow through the hose will be even less. The symptoms you were trying to get rid of will grow worse, not better.

For those who are not weak, regular purification can keep them strong. Taking some time out on a regular basis for purification can help to keep you young and fit. It can be done at the change of season. Or it can be done more frequently such as once a week. Either way, a purification diet can give the digestion a rest and let it do some internal housecleaning. It will also cause some weight to be lost in many people.

Digestive toxins are the basis for disease. They block the intelligent life force from manifesting and flowing through the body. It is important to eliminate them. It is even more important to prevent them from forming. Enhancing digestion is one way of preventing them. Eating according to the principles of Enlightened Nutrition is another. Here are some suggestions for preventing the formation of digestive toxins.

Maximize Your Knowledge

Avoiding *Ama*

In order to minimize the formation of digestive toxins, I recommend the following:

- Optimize digestive power. (See the previous chapter. This is **the** most important recommendation.)
- Take only the purest and freshest food.
- Eat predominantly vegetarian food.
- Eat organically-produced food.
- Avoid genetically-engineered food.
- Avoid "sale" food that is old.
- Do not eat burned or rotting foods. Avoid microwave ovens.

Other ways of purifying do exist. Fasting is one example. The problem with fasting is that it is quite jarring to the system. When impurities come out quickly, the process can be unpleasant. Headaches, digestive problems, and spaciness are just a few of the problems. Doing things gradually has great benefit in that it doesn't disrupt your life. Gradual purification can be done with a special diet taken once weekly. It can also be done with special herbal formulations. Both of these are outlined below.

Experiment #5

The Liquid Diet Experience

This principle of *ama* is so important that another experiment to help bring home the point is provided. This experiment is also a method of purification, so it can be used on a regular basis (once a week) to help keep digestion strong and *ama* levels low.

Required Materials:
A Blender

Method:
Choose a day when your physical and mental demands are not great. A weekend day that is not over-scheduled is usually best. Take only liquids on this day. This does not mean only water. This means a liquid diet. Juices are allowed. Milk is allowed. Soups are allowed. Soups should be pureed in the blender to liquefy their contents, unless they are just a thin broth. Even rice and bean dishes can be liquefied in this manner, by adding some hot water in the blender.

- Try to avoid tomato soup and tomato-based products (like V-8 juice).
- Try to avoid taking too much breakfast the following day. (You don't have to "make up" for any food you missed.)

Write down your experiences in the evening of the day *after* your liquid diet.

Obviously if you are an insulin-dependent diabetic or on medication that is influenced by what you eat such as warfarin (Coumadin), you should not undertake this exercise. Many of my patients who have done this exercise found it very revealing. Here are some of their observations:

"I thought I would not be able to do this experiment. The thought of fasting for a day kept coming to me. But this was different. I was surprised how little hunger I had during the day. It seemed that if I had any hunger, I would just take some juice, and that would be all I needed for hours. It made me realize how much I tend to overeat."
— *Jill S., Bank Clerk*

"I noticed the next day that I felt lighter. I needed less sleep and woke up feeling very refreshed and energetic. I really like the feeling and plan on doing it again."
— *Andrea S., Manager*

"When I got hungry in the evening, I took a thick soup made of rice, cooked zucchini, and cooked red lentils all blended with some hot water. It wasn't like taking a regular meal, and I did take a large bowl, but I was able to make it through to the next day without any problem. I didn't notice much the next day, except that I was very hungry at breakfast and lunch."
— *Brendon L., Banker*

"I felt so clear the next day after the liquid diet. It seemed as if a fog had lifted. I definitely felt like the break helped my digestion, too."
— *Amy Z., Student*

Purification has many facets and can take different avenues. This liquid fast can allow digestion to have a break, so that it can start to digest some of the toxins that have built up in the body. But purification must also take place on the level of the mind. Old habits of the mind keep you stuck accumulating *ama*. Releasing these old stresses allows the mind to purify and habits to change.

Nothing is as purifying to the mind as meditation. I consistently observe that when my patients start practicing an effortless, mantra-based meditation, old habits fall away. Some people "forget" to smoke. Some people "lose the taste" for alcohol. As the mind purifies itself of old associations and old stresses, behavior changes for the better. Eating habits improve naturally. Meditation is a major purifier.

Other sophisticated methods of purification exist. Small packets of intelligence can direct the body to clean up its act. The instructions for this process are contained in the complex molecules of certain plants. These herbs impart their intelligence to the body and direct it to release accumulated toxins. I caution readers to consult with their healthcare providers before starting any herbal regimen, particularly if they are taking prescription medications.

Sometimes the colon is the main source of toxin buildup. This is the case if constipation is present. If the trash is not taken out on a daily basis, it starts to rot. This can become a source of toxins for the body, even if diet is pure and digestion is efficient. If bowel movements do not occur daily, then the breeding ground for toxins is formed.

Again, I caution not to take herbal formulas without consultation. However, using herbal formulas is better than just taking a laxative. Laxatives can be harsh and can actually weaken the colon. They can make the colon muscles lax and cause constipation when overused. The knowledge of combining herbs can mitigate side effects and eliminate this problem.

Unfortunately, our culture has become "pill-oriented." In the rush to accomplish so much and have a full life, health is too often relegated to the nutritional supplements that can be popped into one's mouth. While I could present some herbal formulas, they work best in conjunction with diet. In fact, diet is usually all that is necessary to correct constipation.

Maximize Your Knowledge

Correcting Constipation with Diet

1. Avoid salty foods such as cheeses.
2. Take 2-4 soaked prunes (soaked in water over night) with 2-4 soaked figs in the morning with breakfast.
3. Avoid meat.
4. Take brown rice with at least one meal of the day.
5. Take 1 tsp psyllium husk powder (available at health food stores) with lassi or yogurt and water; put in the blender (1 part yogurt to 3 parts water).

Since diet is key to success with purification, I will present some elements of a purification diet. This is not your ultimate diet, as it is to be used for limited time and is quite restrictive. But certainly some of the principles we have encountered thus far are incorporated into it. This diet works well with herbal formulas for purification. Please note that you may lose some weight with this diet. Therefore, if your weight is low or you are weak, this diet is not for you. If purification is something new to you, you may want to try it only for a week at most to start.

The strategy behind the diet is to avoid foods that can create toxins. This is the reason for taking a light diet. The other aspect of purification is to avoid extremes in taste. For those who have large amounts of digestive toxins and who are carrying a lot of extra weight, the diet can be continued for up to six weeks at a time.

In order to keep the diet from becoming too much of a straightjacket, I will describe the basics first. From that, you can vary the contents of the diet within the guidelines. Remember that purification can induce mild discomfort as the toxins move out. Do not feel that you cannot tolerate the diet at the first sign of some energy swings or cravings.

Note that this diet is very similar to the macrobiotic diet. Macrobiotics was made popular in this country by Michio Kushi. Kushi drew on the teachings of Osawa, one of the foremost proponents of Traditional Japanese Medicine. The diet below varies only with the addition a diluted yogurt drink (lassi). This drink is optional, but does have some important purifying effects, as well as restoring beneficial bacteria to the gut. Milk products are not a common part of the Japanese culture and therefore not part of the macrobiotic diet *per se*. They are thought to be heavy and clogging. However, the process of diluting with water and adding spices can counter this concern.

First, the basics of the diet. Lunch should be the main meal of the day. It should be composed as follows:

LUNCH
1) 25% whole grain
2) 25% beans (small legumes such as red lentil or moong dahl preferred)

*3) 50% fresh vegetables, lightly sautéed or
   steamed (minimum 2 per meal)*
4) Spices to aid digestion
*5) Lassi (diluted yogurt drink to aid the
   intestinal flora)*

I will explain more about the lassi a bit later. It plays an important role, both in terms of purification and in terms of nutrition. It should only be taken during the daytime, not at night. Dinner is as follows:

DINNER
1) 25% whole grain
*2) 25% bean (small legumes such as red lentil or
   moong dahl preferred)*
*3) 50% fresh vegetables, lightly sautéed or
   steamed (minimum 2 per meal)*
4) Spices to aid digestion

Last is breakfast. Breakfast, actually, is optional. If you have hunger, you should take it. If you're not hungry, do not take it. Breakfast should be as follows:

BREAKFAST
1) Stewed apple or pear (see recipe Chapter 3)
*2) Whole-grain cereal (oatmeal, basmati rice)
   with almond milk and raisins*

And for those who get hungry in the afternoon and need a snack to make it to dinnertime:

SNACK
*1) Organic fruit (grapes, pears, pomegranates,
   papaya are best); OR*
2) Soaked Figs

For helping the detoxification process, a spice water should be sipped daily until 6 PM. The recipe for this as well as for lassi and some easy grain and bean dishes follow. The spice water is a very important part of the process. It is a very potent purifier that doesn't cost much money and greatly enhances the process.

Here are the basic rules for the purification diet:

- Food must be freshly prepared, preferably in your own home.
- Do not use frozen or canned foods.
- Do not consume any leftovers (food that has been cooked and not consumed within four to six hours or one to two hours for vegetables).
- Use organically grown food whenever possible.
- Avoid meat.
- No oil or heavy food preparation such as fried foods, cream sauces, and heavy desserts.
- No raw vegetables or salads.
- No breads, except unleavened breads such as chapatis.
- No dairy products except lassi.
- No cold water or ice.
- No alcohol.
- No caffeinated drinks.
- No vinegar-containing substances such as catsup, mustard, pickles, olives, relish, etc.
- Avoid chilies, hot peppers, and jalapeños.

This seems like an arduous task, but anyone can put up with these restrictions for a week. So, if you need to purify, give this diet a try for just seven days. You will be surprised at how much difference this one week makes. To make it easier, I give some more detail about the diet.

One of the most important grains is rice. Basmati rice is particularly revered in Ayurvedic Medicine, as it is thought to be the least likely to create imbalances.

*** See Recipe for Health – Basmati Rice in Appendix II ***

Enjoying: Beans

Beans are the main source of protein in the purification diet. Beans also provide important nutrients such as iron. In fact, ¾ cup of lentils has more iron than 4 oz. of steak. Beans are notorious for creating problems with flatulence. This is a sign that the beans were not well-digested. Beans must be cooked properly. For the purification diet, the small beans made into soups are the best (red lentils, moong dahl). Other beans or peas may be taken on a limited basis if they do not create digestive disturbance. Here are some rules for making sure beans are fully digested:

1. Always check beans for pebbles.
2. Always rinse beans before cooking. The helps reduce beans' main source of flatulence and indigestibility: oligosaccharides. Rinse until no more froth is created by stirring the beans in the water.
3. Simmer beans in fresh water—never in the rinse water.
4. After bringing to a boil, partially cover and reduce heat to simmer. It is important to simmer the beans, not boil them. When boiled they become tough and hard to digest.
5. Always skim off any foam that comes to the top. During cooking, a foamy scum made of starches, proteins, and minerals can form on the top. This is where some of the oligosaccharides reside, and skimming them off greatly increases the digestibility of beans.
6. Never add cold water to cooking beans. They may stop the process and cause the beans to become hard. If you need more water, add boiling water from a kettle.
7. Never add salt, baking soda, tomatoes, or lemon juice to simmer beans. Any shifts in acidity or alkalinity will cause the surface of the beans to harden and prevent further absorption of water, making them hard, tough, and difficult to digest.
8. Never take beans without spices or oil. Beans need spice to stimulate digestion. These should be added at the end of the cooking process. A small amount of ghee or olive oil will help to counter the drying effects of beans. Fry your spices briefly in oil in order to bring out their flavor.
9. Never undercook beans. Undercooking will guarantee indigestibility. When adequately cooked, beans will often have a soupy consistency.

Beans and legumes form an important part of the purification diet (or any diet for that matter). Several tricks can help you to enjoy this natural source of protein. If these rules are followed beans can become an exciting part of the diet, not something relegated to a picnic now and then. Indian cooking is famous for its *dahls*. These are lentils made with spices and oil and cooked to a thick pureed consistency. Remember: It is not *dahl* unless it contains spices and oil and has a liquid consistency.

** See Recipe for Health - Moong Dahl in Appendix II **

I commented that oil is a necessary part of *dahls*, but I haven't said much about this important aspect of the diet. Oil is important in the diet, as the body cannot manufacture all the substances the body requires without essential oils in the diet. This is one area that tends to be overdone in the American diet. Therefore, I have included some information on it as follows.

Enjoying: Oils

So much confusion exists in the area of oils. The American diet is far too burdened with fats and oils, and this has laid the foundation for arguments as to what the best oil is. Often ignored in the debate is the importance of quantity and quality of oil. The major culprit in the U.S. is quantity. People do not realize that even the leanest cut of meat is more than 30% fat in terms of calories. In between the little muscle fibers are fat deposits that the muscle used for energy storage. These micro-globules of fat are simply not visible, but serve to make greasing the pan you fry your hamburger in unnecessary.

The purification diet contains no meat. It contains no oils, and the body does need some essential oils in the diet. So adding some oil to *dahls* or sautéing spices in some oil to put on vegetables is important. What is the best oil?

First, the oil must be organic. Many pesticides are soluble in lipid and are carried in the oil fraction of the plant. Non-organic oils can be a concentrated form of pesticide contamination.

Second, the oil should not be genetically engineered. Here is another reason for buying organic. Genetic engineering is a huge laboratory experiment on the ecosystem and has already been shown to cause dangers. The ramifications of toying with the molecular basis of life cannot be guaranteed to be safe.

Third, do not use lard or rapeseed oil. Lard does not fit well with a vegetarian diet (it has the wrong energy), and it is also a carrier of pesticides. The ancients noted that rapeseed oil easily became toxic when heated.

Enjoying: Oils (cont.)

Knowing this, do not take canola oil. Canola oil is **Can**adian rapeseed oil. It has been cleverly marketed under a new name. Unfortunately, the vast majority of it is genetically engineered and is not organic. Furthermore, even if it were organic, the inherent qualities of rapeseed oil make its use precarious.

The best oil to use is organic extra virgin, cold pressed olive oil. Refined oils are damaging to the body. Extra virgin means it has not been processed. The ancient seers knew that oils can be heating to the system and can be heavy to digest. Olive oil has a more cooling property. Rapeseed oil has one of the hottest. Coconut oil is also cooling in nature but is very heavy and hard to digest.

The other oil that is excellent for the body (in moderation) is ghee, or clarified butter. Most people think that butter is the worst oil because it contains saturated fats; however, when the milk solids are removed and the pure oil consumed, it becomes much more benign.

Ghee is composed of very short-chained fatty acids. This is what makes it different from other saturated fats. Other oils and fats have long carbon chains (from 16 to 18 in length) that compose the backbone of the oil. The main fatty acid in ghee is butyric acid, which has only four carbons. These short chains are less likely to be involved in oxidative damage (free radical problems). They make cell walls more fluid and flexible than the long chain fatty acids. Ghee, taken is small amounts, doesn't increase cholesterol either. It is cooling in nature, so it makes one of the best oils, in moderation.

Just as it is important that your olive oil be organic, it is essential that your ghee be made from organic butter. Otherwise, it can be carry pesticides and other harmful substances. I provide a recipe for making your own ghee, as it is quite simple.

Do not just use only ghee for everything. It is best to have variety in the diet. Without it, the chances of imbalance are greater and the chance that you will tire of the diet is much greater also.

** See Recipe for Health - Ghee in Appendix II **

Spices are an important component of Enlightened Nutrition and also of this purification diet. Exploring the intense tastes that spices offer a meal is one of the exciting parts of eating. Culinary expertise requires a detailed knowledge of spices. It is never too early to start exploring.

Enjoying: Spices

Spice your food at each meal. This helps the digestive process and, of course, adds flavor. Spices to consider during your purification diet:

- **Indian spices:** *Turmeric, cumin, coriander, fennel.*
- **Italian spices:** *Oregano, basil, parsley, rosemary.*
- **English spices:** *Thyme, mint, sage.*
- **Other:** *Ginger root, black pepper (both in small quantities).*
- **Salt:** Use sparingly. Prefer rock salt.

To spice your vegetables: After steaming the vegetables, you may add a mixture of 1-2 teaspoons of oil sautéed with spices. To prepare, heat 1-2 teaspoons of oil over medium low heat in a sauce pan. First add seeds (like cumin) and fry gently until golden brown. Then add any of the powdered spices. Pour this mixture over the vegetables, adding fresh herbs such as parsley or cilantro at the very end. As an alternative to steaming, lightly sauté vegetables in your spice mixture.

Spices make up an important part of the cleansing effect of the purification diet. In order to enhance this, drinking a spice water throughout the day can help.

Maximize Your Knowledge

Spice Water Recipe

Drink all day long until 6 PM during purification diet.
Boil 1 quart of spring water for 5 minutes. Pour into a thermos. Add the following spices in WHOLE seed form:

¼ tsp cumin seeds
¼ tsp coriander seeds
½ tsp fennel seeds

Sip on the spice water throughout the day every half hour or so.

You may drink other water during the day according to thirst, but try to drink all the spice water by the end of the day. However, do not drink the spice water after 6 PM or its diuretic effect may keep you awake at night.

The spice water must be made fresh every day.

When you are pursuing a purification diet, it is important to avoid sugar. When you need something sweet, take a fig or some fresh sweet fruit (mango is excellent). You can use a little honey, but this should be at most two teaspoons per day. Avoid other sweeteners such as corn syrup or brown rice syrup or molasses during this time, as well. Remember: Almost anyone can do this diet for seven days if you simply remind yourself that it is not forever. Furthermore, the experience you have exploring new grains and new ways of spicing things will make it interesting. That, combined with your experience of how you feel at the end of the week, will make it all the easier to do it the next time.

Drinking your spice water during this purification period is one of the most important parts of the process. The spice water helps with the flushing of toxins. It stimulates the internal housecleaning process. Taking some extra fluid at this time helps the body to flush things out, and making sure you get your spice water in between meals is a way to assure this happens.

One other important purifying agent in the process is lassi. Lassi is a dilute yogurt drink. It is the major source of vitamin B12 in the purification diet. It alters the intestinal flora, so that the gut health is restored. This helps with both absorption and assimilation of nutrients. It particularly aids the large colon, where many of the problems with health originate (at least according to the ancient seers).

The lactose and other factors that often cause people trouble with dairy have been "predigested" by the bacteria in the yogurt. Most of the problems people have with yogurt are because it is taken in concentrated form, not in the dilute form of lassi. Store-bought yogurt is heavy and hard to digest. It is old and more sour than homemade yogurt. These factors are what cause it to be shunned by many. By making homemade lassi, most of these problems are avoided.

*** See Recipe for Health — Yogurt in Appendix II ***

*** See Recipe for Health — Lassi in Appendix II ***

I mentioned before that it is not advisable during purification to eat yeasted bread products. Yeasts cause many people problems. They aggravate digestion. They make bread harder to digest. They can cause a buildup of toxins. They can also cause some heating effect. In addition, yeasts form gases that can be hard on the colon. Much has been made of the systemic candidiasis issue. This is the effect that yeast can have on the entire system. It occurs when digestion is weak and can't eliminate the yeast. This then forms a toxic type of *ama* that causes an almost allergic type of reaction. The diet that is recommended to fight this condition is basically a purification diet. Unfortunately, many people get trapped into thinking this is the way one "should" eat. After purification is done, the diet needs to broaden and be less restrictive. Digestion should be strengthened so that the situation will not recur.

Understanding digestion and the fact that it can be strengthened or weakened puts such diets in a new light. Once the situation is addressed at the root cause (weak digestion), then purifying or restrictive diets do not need to be continued for the rest of one's life. This is the beauty of a deep understanding of how the body functions. Altering the digestion can cure the situation. Otherwise, one must constantly restrict the diet and avoid one food or another.

For those who are used to taking bread with meals or consuming large quantities of pasta, some unleavened bread can be taken during the purification diet. While some health food stores carry unleavened breads, you may find yourself having to make your own. It is not as difficult as it sounds. For those of you who are ambitious, I present a recipe for the traditional Indian unleavened bread called chapatis.

*** See Recipe for Health — Unleavened Bread in Appendix II ***

I have presented ways of purification that combine both spices, spice waters, and diet. The concept of purification is foreign to Western medicine. But the experience of seeing a tongue coated with undigested material is not foreign at all. Knowing that digestion is not always optimal and that it can be improved necessitates a fresh look at purification. It is something that is needed on a regular basis. Avoiding the buildup of toxins is key to health and longevity. Understanding this paves the way to your ultimate diet.

* 7 *

Food as Medicine

Let food be thy medicine.
— Hippocrates

Judy D. reports to her physician's office for the results of her colonoscopy. She had been diagnosed with ulcerative colitis four years ago. She awaits the results with some anxiety. She has not been following her doctor's orders. In fact, she has not been taking any of her medication. After two years of struggling with her condition and the side effects of the drugs she was taking, she decided she had had enough.

Approaching 40 years of age, she felt she could make some decisions on her own. "The drugs were causing me as much problem as the disease. I just felt like I was getting nowhere fast." She decided to take matters into her own hands and stopped her medications. This is certainly something no physician would recommend. She instead sought out the help of an Ayurvedic physician.

"I knew this had something to do with diet. In what way, I did not know. I knew it was connected, but I did not know how." She learned the basic principles of balancing the body's physiological functions or *doshas*. She was given a diet to decrease fire or *pitta* dosha, as her inflammation in the colon was a sign of *pitta* and *ama*. She immediately noticed a change in her bowel movements.

At first, she had a decrease in the number of bowel movements from eight to ten per day down to three to five. Then she noticed the bowel movements started to become more well-formed. Her diarrhea went away. Eventually, after trying some herbal formulas, she found a diet that could allow her to have a normal life again with normal bowel movements. She did not tell her doctor what she was doing. Now it was time again for her checkup and her colonoscopy results.

"I have some good news for you," her specialist begins. "Your colon shows no signs of ulceration. In fact, the wall of the colon looks normal. The medicine must be working."

"I have some news for you," she replies. "I'm not taking any medication." Her doctor's mouth drops open.

"How can that be?" he asks. She tries to describe her newfound diet and the concepts of balance. She is met with disbelief. Her doctor concludes, "Sometimes this happens as we grow older. I know you think it is related to diet. But we really have no evidence that diet makes a difference in this disease."

Judy's story points to the contrast between East and West. For the Eastern physician, diet is intimate to life, balance, and health. To the allopathic physician, diet is unrelated to most disease. By now, if you have been doing these experiments, you have begun to feel the impact food and diet have on the body. To bring home the point, I provide yet another experiment in self-discovery.

Experiment #6

The Salt Experiment

This experiment can be undertaken as a "thought" experiment by those who are hypertensive or are otherwise salt-sensitive. It should be especially avoided by those with heart problems and heart failure. Many of you may have already by chance had this experience, in which case you can simply reflect back and write down your experience.

Required Materials:
- Potato chips
- Pretzels (salted)
- Mozzarella cheese
- Rye bread

Method:
The strategy is to experience the effects of having one's body exposed to one prevailing taste. In order to do this, the first two meals of the day will be predominant in salty taste. For this one-time-only experiment, try the following:

1) Eat only potato chips for breakfast.
2) If you need a mid-morning snack, take only salted pretzels.
3) You may drink as much water as you need, but do not take any other flavored liquid.
4) For lunch have a sandwich with mozzarella cheese on rye bread. (You can have some lettuce and Mayonnaise on it, if you wish.)
5) For a mid-afternoon snack take pretzels.

Write down your experience.

Many people have "overdosed" on salt before in their lives and don't have to go through this experiment to know its effects. Whether you do this experiment by memory or by the instructions above, try to consider the following questions as you reflect on your experience:

- How does the experience of salty taste change over the day?

- Why might it be difficult to take salty taste first thing in the morning?

- Does the body start to favor tastes other than salty after some time? If so, which tastes?

- Does plain water satisfy the thirst that the salt creates? If not, why not?

- Could you survive on a salt-based diet? Why would you desire anything else?

I will discuss the deeper aspects of these questions and give some insights from the ancient seers. Before doing so, here are some of the experiences of our patients who were bold enough to follow through with this experiment.

"Salty taste is the last thing I ever crave in the morning, even if I wake up hungry. It was difficult to get down more than a couple of the potato chips."
— *Tori G., Beautician*

"By the time mid-afternoon came around, I was dying for something sweet. Some fruit juice or candy ... anything with a sweet taste. I wasn't even really hungry. I just needed something else to counter that salty taste."
— *Ellen A., Homemaker*

"It was a strange day. To tell you the truth, besides being a bit thirsty, I didn't notice too much. I wouldn't want to eat this way every day, but just one day didn't impact me much. I guess I am

used to taking a lot of salt in my diet anyway ...”
— *Harold M., Retired Autoworker*

“I notice right after 'breakfast' that I needed something sweet. It just got worse as the day went on. Each 'meal' became less appetizing. I just wanted some sugar to balance out all the salt.”
— *Jan. P., Massage Therapist*

“I have done this once or twice in the past — where I got cravings for salt and then binged on it. Then I would flip and get cravings for sugar. If I took enough sweets then I would flip back. This was not so bad, because I did not start out with the salt cravings. But it did seem that by the afternoon, I was wanting something sweet to balance out all the salty taste. I didn't need sugar. I would have settled for some fruit even. Just something with a cooling, soothing taste.”
— *Kelly K., Student*

“I noticed I ate a lot less than usual and still didn't have cravings. I got sick of the pretzels very fast. I didn't get particularly thirsty, but I sure was bored with the pretzels. I would have settled for a doughnut or something sweet instead.”
— *Edward M., Photographer*

One of the fundamental principles of ancient medical systems is that the body is intelligent. You don't have to think to form a scab, heal it, and turn it back into skin again. The body is smart enough to do this on its own. Likewise, the body is always seeking to maintain balance. When too much acid is taken in, it flushes acid out through the kidney. The body communicates its needs through desire—a desire for this taste or a craving for this food. Each reflects the body's attempt to reach an equilibrium and to balance out some factor, either physical or mental.

Taste communicates the qualities of the food or substance. These qualities have a direct effect on the balance and functioning of the body. Take a diet that is loaded with salt, and immediately the body will start craving something to balance it. Take a diet high in acid, and the urine becomes acidic, as the body seeks to eliminate the excess.

The ancient seers cognized the effects that different tastes have on the physiology. In doing so, they picked the language of nature to describe what they observed. While they described things in terms of fire, water, and earth, they were not so naïve as to think that the body was actually made of these things. Their perceptions were on a much more subtle level. They may have been actually cognizing the fundamental qualities of the subatomic particles that compose the body. Regardless, their description gives a new language with which to describe balance and homeostasis.

What is the impact of a substance on the body? How does it create balance or imbalance? To understand this in detail, some new terms need to be introduced.

THE INSIDE SCOOP

The Doshas

The ancient rishis who cognized Ayurveda saw that subtle energies underlying physical creation had a five-fold nature. They described these vibrational qualities in the language of nature:

Air   Space   Fire   Water   Earth

These occur at a level that is not yet manifested in physical creation. These vibrations or energies guide the formation of physical existence. The qualities combine in the body to form physiological principles — that which guides the physiological functioning. These combinations are called **doshas** and are described below:

Vata: Composed of air and space, this dosha is subtle and diffuse like air. Just as the wind moves things about in an invisible way, so too does vata. It is responsible for movement in the body. Respiration, peristalsis (movement of food through the digestive track), elimination, and movement of information from the nerves to the brain are all under the influence of vata. Its primary functions are MOVEMENT and COMMUNICATION.

When vata is out of balance and becomes excessive, the nervous system is affected, movement in the body becomes less coordinated, and the emotions become changeable. The stress on the nervous system creates anxiety and fear, and when severe one actually "shakes" physically. Typical vata imbalances are insomnia, anxiety disorder, irritable bowel syndrome, PMS, constipation, and conditions that result from the drying effects of "wind": dry skin, dandruff, and eczema.

Pitta: *Composed of fire and a small portion of water, this dosha is hot in nature. Just as fire transforms things and creates heat, pitta dosha is responsible for the "fires" of the body. That means it is responsible for metabolism both on the cellular level and on the level of the body as a whole. Pitta transforms things, and so it is no surprise that the liver is one of its primary organs. Pitta is responsible for that aspect of digestion that is involved in breaking down food and transforming it into something the body can use. Pittas main functions are* **DIGESTION, METABOLISM,** *and* **TRANSFORMATION.**

When pitta is out of balance, these functions tend to be affected resulting in such conditions as heartburn, indigestion, and high cholesterol. When this dosha is in excess it makes things too "hot" and creates inflammation, infections, and redness in areas of the body. This can result in such things as ulcers, inflammatory bowel disease, skin rashes, acne, or heart disease.

Kapha: *Composed of earth and water, it creates the heavy structure of the body and is responsible for its lubrication, strength, endurance, and water balance. Kapha regulates the physical growth of the body. It lubricates the joints and the linings of the lungs and the cerebral spinal fluid that surrounds the brain. Kapha's main functions are* **STRUCTURE, LUBRICATION,** *and* **STRENGTH** *or* **IMMUNITY.**

When kapha is out of balance, immunity is weak, and congestion predominates. Typical kapha disorders include sinusitis, colds, flus, and water retention. Conditions that result from excess "structure" or kapha include diabetes, congestive heart failure, and tumors.

Keeping the doshas in balance means the basic functions of the body are in balance.

Utilizing these ancient concepts can help us understand the results of the salt experiment. For most people who do the experiment, any craving for salt taste passes quickly and is replaced by a craving for something to balance out the salty taste. Salt is heating in nature. Like salt in a wound, it burns. Sweet taste is cooling in nature. It counters salt. This understanding allows our next principle to be introduced:

Principle #5: The body constantly seeks to maintain balance.

The body's striving for balance is what forces one to crave a particular taste or food. It satisfies some need in the body (or mind). Taste is the mechanism through which the qualities of a substance and its effects are known. Certain tastes increase the actions of certain processes within the body and increase certain *doshas*. Others decrease the actions of those processes. Knowing this, the balance and the functioning of the body can be altered toward healthful living. Knowledge from the seers can help put the pieces of this puzzle together.

In macrobiotics salt is considered very *Yang*. It is active, heating, and dynamic. The body strives to balance this with foods that are cooling. Sweet is very *yin* in nature and is quite the opposite in qualities. In this ancient system, it is no wonder that cravings for sweet follow excess salt intake. Sweet and salty are not the only tastes. Each has its actions and influence on balance. The ancients described these effects in detail.

THE INSIDE SCOOP

Tastes and the Body's Balance

Here is what the ancients understood to be the effect of each taste in terms of action of the food on the physiology:

SWEET: Anabolic (that is, it builds up the body). Consolidating and cooling. It cools and soothes the body. It increases lubrication in the body. "Sweet taste tonifies, balances and moderates. It is used to tonify deficiency and to stop pain." Remember: The body uses mucous to lubricate. Mucous is composed of carbohydrate chains or sugars chained together. Mucous soothes dryness and cools inflammation. In the Ayurvedic system it increases kapha and soothes vata and pitta.

SOUR: Heating, anabolic, and moisturizing. Remember: Sour things are acidic. Acid is burning or heating. When you put something sour in the mouth, it tends to increase saliva. In Chinese Medicine sour taste generates fluids and yin (such as moisturizing substances). In Ayurvedic Medicine it is said to decrease and soothe the dryness of vata, to heat pitta, and to make kapha more watery (that is, aggravate pitta and kapha).

SALTY: Heating. Draws water into it, so it is anabolic. In the Chinese system salt is said to soften hardness and help "downward flow" in the body. Remember: Salt in a wound burns. Its heat counters the coldness of the wind (vata, in the Ayurvedic system) and increases fire (pitta). Salt draws water to it like a salt crystal thrown on an icy sidewalk (increases kapha).

PUNGENT: Catabolic. Heating. Dispersing. In Chinese Medicine "The pungent taste scatters and is used to expel pathogenic factors." Remember: Pungent tastes are those hot tastes like chilies and ginger. They burn through the mucous (decreasing kapha) and create heartburn (increased pitta). Because they are so hot, they dry things out (aggravate vata).

BITTER: Catabolic. Cooling. Hardening. "The bitter taste clears Heat, sedates and hardens. It clears Damp-Heat and it subdues Rebellious Qi." In the Ayurvedic system it increases vata — decreases pitta and kapha. Remember: Bitter is cooling (decreases fire and inflammation) and drying (dries out wet moisture).

ASTRINGENT: Catabolic. Hardening. Astringent taste is drying and composed of the elements air and earth in the Ayurvedic system of thought. Astringent taste is found in beans and foods like pomegranate and lemon that make your mouth pucker or feel dry.

How does all this get applied? This understanding paves the way for food to be used as medicine. Food, over time, affects the balance and physiological functioning of the body. Food has more than just biochemical value. It conveys its qualities to the body. Bitter foods are catabolic. They lighten the body. Light foods lighten the body. Sweet foods are anabolic. They are heavy and body-building. Heavy foods make the body heavier. Spicy hot foods add flame to the body; in excess, they "inflame" it. Cold foods cool the digestion and make the digestion run "cold," so that it does not burn effectively. Dry foods dry the body.

The subtle qualities of food are lost on most of us. Few have developed their awareness to the point where they experience the impact of the qualities of food. Qualities are more complex than just hot or cold, heavy or light, wet or dry. Take the quality of bitterness, for example. Bitterness contains within it dryness and coldness and lightness. Bitter foods impart all of these qualities to the body. The action of any substance, when understood completely in terms of its qualities, can predict its effects on the body. Bitter substances will cool the body, decreasing heat or inflammation in the body, decreasing moisture and mass, and making the body drier and lighter. How can this knowledge be used medicinally?

Suppose we have a condition whose essence is hot and moist. What sort of condition might this be? Consider a pimple or small boil. A boil has moisture in it. It is an accumulation of moisture and substance, of pus. It is also an inflamed area of the body. Thus, it has both elements of *kapha* (earth/moisture) and *pitta* (fire/inflammation). In the Chinese system it has the characteristics of *damp heat*. In allopathic medicine, this can be treated with an antibiotic, such as tetracycline. Tetracycline has a bitter quality to it. Most antibiotics are intensely bitter, if one tastes them rather than just swallowing the pill whole. This quality is imparted to the body on all levels. Because it is a refined substance, a single chemical structure, this bitterness is extremely concentrated.

The effects on the body of tetracycline's bitterness can be understood in terms of its side effects, caused by its intensity. In 10 percent of people tetracycline causes gastrointestinal irritation resulting in nausea, vomiting, anorexia, flatulence, diarrhea, or dryness of mouth. Bitterness has a drying effect. The stomach protects itself from the acid it uses to digest food with mucus. Mucus is a *kapha* or *phlegm* substance. Bitter decreases *kapha* or *phlegm/damp heat*. Intense bitterness cuts through and decreases mucus. Thus, the mucus lining the stomach will be disturbed, and the stomach will be exposed to acid. This can cause nausea, vomiting, anorexia, flatulence, and diarrhea. Tetracycline can also suppress bone growth because bitter is *catabolic*. It consumes structure and makes it lighter. Other side effects are light-headedness and dizziness. Bitterness makes lightness. The list of tetracycline's side effects is very long, but those most commonly encountered can be understood from knowing the underlying qualities of its taste. Is there a way to impart the qualities of tetracycline to the body without the side effects?

On a continuum of medicinal substances, herbs are less potent than antibiotics, but they also induce fewer side effects. Goldenseal is a very bitter herb that is considered to have antibiotic, antibacterial, and antiseptic properties. It is prescribed in various forms in herbal medicine for inflammatory and infectious conditions. The fact that it is bitter gives a clue to its use. It also gives a clue to some of the precautions that should be taken in its use, as propounded by expert herbalists. It should not be used in people with disorders such as vertigo (dizziness), emaciation, and chronic debility. Again bitterness makes lightness and can make for light-headedness. It lightens the body and will make the emaciated worse. Yet, it is not as fraught with side effects as is tetracycline, because it is not as purely bitter. It is buffered by the other substances within the plant. However, it must usually be taken longer than tetracycline in order to have an effect, as its onset of action is also much longer.

Further along this continuum of medicinal substances are spices. It is logical that if we want to avoid the side effects of herbs, we can use spices. Spices are much better tolerated than antibiotics or bitter herbs. Bitter spices can be used to gently convey the same effect to the body. Coriander is an example of a bitter spice that we might choose instead of a bitter herb.

Finally, at the extreme end of the spectrum, bitter foods can convey the qualities of lightness and dryness to the body. They too can have anti-inflammatory effects. But the duration of administration is much longer — measured in months often, rather than days, as is the case with antibiotics. Compared to drugs and herbs, food has almost no side effects. In this manner, food can be medicine and can be used preventively. Before the boil erupts, the *kapha* and *pitta* excess (or *damp heat*) in the body can be detected by the experienced alternative physician. In this setting, prescribing the right food and spices can rebalance the body and prevent the boil from ever developing. Herein lies a vast field of study in the art of prevention. Contained in this field of study is an exact description of the effects of foods on the body, and their utilization as medicine. By taking foods to rebalance the body *before* disease arises, food is raised to its ultimate purpose: preventive medicine perfected.

In introducing Ayurveda to the West, the concept of body types was emphasized. This was in contrast to the Western medical approach that treats every person the same way. It was a refreshing reminder that "one man's meat is another man's poison." Tailoring diet and herbal recommendations to the individual was a welcomed change. Likewise, Ayurveda emphasizes understanding "who this individual is." Understanding one's body type in terms of vata, pitta, or kapha gives this unique approach a more human, caring approach.

We all have all three doshas, just in different proportions. Most of us are dual dosha types — that is, we are a combination composed predominantly of two of the doshas. Vata-pitta or pitta-kapha are examples. Someone who is very lightweight and moves quickly (like the wind) is an example of a vata type. Someone who is heavy and grounded and moves slowly is an example of a kapha type. A fiery redhead is an example of a pitta type.

Taking a diet tailored to our particular body type makes intuitive sense to us. It is part of the reason for the success of such diets as the Blood Type diet. Remember, though, that the qualities inherent in a diet tend to influence the balance in the body. For someone who is in perfect balance, diet should be based on one's body type. But who among us can claim to be in perfect balance?

The real focus and purpose of the following diets is to bring about balance in the doshas. Whatever dosha is out of balance or in excess, that is the dosha-balancing diet that should be taken. A pitta type person can have a vata imbalance and need to address and rebalance vata through diet for some time. A vata type can have a pitta imbalance and need to take some cooling foods to bring things back to equilibrium.

The purpose of the following diets is not to give you a diet for your body type. These diets are rebalancing diets. Like the purification diet, they are for special situations. They are to rebalance. They are *not* the ultimate diet. They draw on the principles of Enlightened Nutrition. They also draw on some of the principles of the purification diet.

They are to be used for two to four months after purification. The understanding in the ancient medical traditions is that purification is undertaken first and then rebalancing. If one attempts to rebalance without purification, *ama* gets in the way. If one attempts purification without rebalancing afterward, then one can risk making imbalances even worse. The purification diet is to be followed in preparation for your ultimate diet.

How do you know what needs rebalancing? Generally, some signs and subtle symptoms can guide your selection of diet. The best solution is to have an alternative physician evaluate your state of balance. From taking the pulse and asking a few key questions, a well-trained physician can assess your balance in a very short period of time. This is an excellent way of knowing what rebalancing diet is best for you. Short of this, the following questions can help to guide your selection.

1) Are your symptoms hot or cold?
In all the ancient medical systems, signs of inflammation or tendency toward inflammation are considered under the category of "hot" symptoms. So ulcers, hot flashes, skin redness or rashes, colitis, heartburn, excessive body heat, excessive anger and passion — these are all considered hot symptoms. Cold symptoms are symptoms of pain, congestion, accumulation of mucous, and cool extremities.

2) Are you strong or weak?
This is a critical question. If you have great strength and great reserve, then a diet that is light and catabolic will not bother you. You tend to suffer from an excess in the balance of the physiology, not a deficiency. If you are thin, weak, and have a tendency toward low energy or frailty, then you need to take an anabolic diet, or one that builds you up. So the choices here are a diet to strengthen or tonify (anabolic) or a diet to lighten and decrease excesses (catabolic).

3) Dry or Moist?

Dry skin, constipation, brittle nails, brittle hair, vaginal dryness, dry eyes, and cracking joints are all signs of dryness in the body. Sinus congestion, oily or mucous-filled stools, oily skin, excessive perspiration, and stiffness are all signs of excessive moisture.

From these characteristics you can then find which tastes to favor in the diet.

Maximize Your Knowledge

Tastes and the Diet

If you are **WEAK,** the predominant taste in the diet should be sweet. The secondary taste in the diet (second most predominant taste) is dependent on whether you have cold or hot symptoms. If you are **HOT**, then the secondary taste should be bitter. The third or tertiary taste is dependent on moisture or dryness in the body. If you are **DRY**, the taste needs to be sour. Use the table below combined with the list of foods to determine how to balance your imbalances with food.

Condition	Predominant Taste	Secondary Taste	Tertiary Taste
Weak, Cold, Dry	Sweet	Salty	Sour
Weak, Hot, Dry	Sweet	Bitter	Sour
Weak, Cold, Moist	Sweet	Salty	Astringent
Weak, Hot, Moist	Sweet	Bitter	Astringent
Strong, Cold, Dry	Bitter	Salty	Sour
Strong, Hot, Dry	Bitter	Bitter	Sour
Strong, Cold, Moist	Bitter	Salty	Astringent
Strong, Hot, Moist	Bitter	Bitter	Astringent

Recall that tastes can sometimes be subtle. We usually think of sweet in terms of desserts and sugared foods. In the natural world, however, grains are sweet. They are carbohydrates, basically, and are essentially composed of natural sugars. Meats are also sweet in nature. What is bitter? Most greens are bitter. What is astringent? Anything that is drying in nature. Most beans are drying in nature, which makes them hard to digest. In order to help you get an understanding of food qualities I have listed predominant tastes in some common foods.

*** See Appendix 1: Ayurvedic Food Properties ***

Admittedly, these considerations can get quite complex. You can drive yourself nuts trying to memorize all of this and create a diet based on your particular health condition. While it is beyond the scope of this book to train you to become an expert in prescribing diet to rebalance, the good news is that most people tend to fall into categories of imbalance. And most of the common patterns can be easily assessed. People tend to fall into one of four categories. That means that I can keep things simple by presenting four basic diets. Recall that after purification, the next step is to rebalance. The direction of rebalancing usually relates to one of four requirements:

1) The need to cool off heat in the body.
Inflammations, tendency towards heartburn, hot emotions, and rashes all dictate that the *Cooling Diet* or *Pitta Pacifying Diet* be taken.

Do you need to cool off? Take a look at the following list of symptoms and count how many of these are present for you.

__Rashes
__Ulcers
__Heartburn
__Blurred vision
__Excessive body heat
__Premature graying or balding
__Anger
__Hostility
__Irritability
__Frustration
__Impatience
__Excessive hunger
__Excessive thirst
__Lack of thirst
__Hot flashes
__Colitis or inflammatory bowel disease
__Canker sores
__Cold sores
__Yellow color of stool, urine, or skin
__Early morning awakenings (and can't get back to sleep)

Now look at the other common patterns.

2) The need to strengthen, soothe, and tonify.

If you are weak or depleted, you may need to start with a tonifying and building diet to get your energy back, build strength, and prepare to purify out old toxins. How do you tell if you are weak? You have fatigue or nervousness predominating your experience. You have no stamina, have multiple symptoms, with the sense that everything is falling apart. You have no endurance, are depressed, have little enthusiasm. You cannot exercise without getting exhausted or without becoming ill. You get many frequent colds and flus. These signs would warn you that you need to tonify and strengthen, rather than undertake purification. For this situation you would take the *Tonification Diet or Vata Pacifying Diet* described below.

How many of the following are present for you?

__Underweight
__Emaciation
__Fatigue (even with sleep)
__Loss of Enthusiasm (depression)
__Insomnia (difficulty falling asleep)
__Constipation
__Constant sense of something being wrong
__Tension headaches
__Intolerance of cold
__Anxiety
__Worry
__Osteoarthritis
__Irritable Bowel Syndrome
__Disturbed elimination
__Menstrual cramps
__Symptoms that keep changing, pains that wander
__Fibromyalgia
__Loss of strength
__Lack of mental clarity

3) The need to reduce, disperse, and continue to purify.

If there has been an accumulation of toxins that is longstanding, then the need is to continue to purify out old *ama*. If you have gained weight and can't lose it, or have a tendency to gain weight and become sluggish, then the *Dispersing & Reducing Diet* or *Kapha Pacifying Diet* is recommended for you.

How many of the following are present for you?

> ___Wake up tired even after a good night's sleep
> ___Feel lethargic
> ___Thick tongue coating
> ___Lack of real hunger
> ___Generalized aches and pains
> ___Feel weary and unenthusiastic
> ___Feel blocked
> ___Sinus congestion
> ___Constipation
> ___Frequent indigestion, bloating, gas
> ___Excessive weight gain
> ___Fluid retention
> ___Unmotivated
> ___Elevated cholesterol
> ___Yeast infections

4) The need to nourish and moisturize without gaining weight.

If dryness predominates the situation, but the individual is not weak, then this requires a different tone to the diet. The *Moisturizing Diet or Light Vata Diet* can help in this situation.

How many of the following are present for you?

> ___Dry skin
> ___Dry eyes
> ___Vaginal dryness
> ___Forgetfulness
> ___Cracking or popping joints
> ___Insomnia (difficulty falling or restless sleep)
> ___Dandruff
> ___Tension headaches
> ___Tendonitis or frequent sprains
> ___Mood swings
> ___Feeling overwhelmed at times
> ___Constipation with dry stools
> ___Heart palpitations

How to select the proper balancing diet.

While you may have checks in all four categories, you will find that one or two categories tend to predominate. If you feel that you have very few symptoms or are fairly balanced, then the last diet (the Light Vata diet) is best for you. If you feel you have checked many in all four categories (greater than five), then start with the purifying or Kapha Diet.

The basic structure of the main meals (lunch and dinner) for each of the four diets is this:

1. *A natural appetizer*
2. *A power grain*
3. *A protein source*
4. *Two vegetable dishes*
5. *A fruit-based dessert*

The basic structure for breakfast is dependent on hunger:

1. *If no hunger: Diet-specific tea.*
2. *Very mild hunger: Diet-specific stewed fruit.*
3. *Moderate hunger: Diet-specific cooked cereal.*
4. *Great hunger: Diet-specific stewed fruit and cooked cereal.*

The most important aspect of each diet is to understand its main principle or rationale. With that in mind, you will soon be able to create your own meals, without having to refer to this book. In the meantime, I present a description of principles.

Maximize Your Knowledge

Cooling or Pitta Pacifying Diet

General Principle: Any food that would burn or irritate if put on an open blister is to be avoided. That means acidic foods like citrus, vinegar, tomatoes, and aged foods like soy sauce, hard cheeses, and old yogurt. It also means salty foods (salt burns in a wound) or spicy-hot foods like chilies, salsa, and pepper. Favor sweet, bitter, and drying or astringent tastes. Remember that oil on a fire causes it to flare and burn more intensely, so take very little oil and no fried foods.

Grains: Quinoa, bulgur wheat, rice (white basmati, Texmati, or jasmine), couscous, pasta (eggless), flat bread made without yeast or baking soda, such as chapatis or tortillas.

High Protein Foods: Moong bean (split or whole), red lentils, green lentils, brown lentils, tofu, pumpkin seeds, almonds (blanched is best). For nonvegetarians: chicken or turkey breast, egg whites.

Vegetables: Winter squashes (such as acorn, butternut, etc.), summer squashes (such as zucchini, yellow squash), fennel, cucumber, asparagus, artichokes, cilantro, all green leafy vegetables (chard, collards, etc.) except spinach (small amounts), sweet potatoes. If you do not have an inflammatory disease you can also take: carrots, green beans, broccoli, cauliflower, cabbage, peas, snow peas, okra, lettuce, brussels sprouts, parsley, bok choy, sweet corn. *Strictly avoid: tomatoes, eggplant, green and red chilies, white potatoes.*

Fruits: Melon, cantaloupe, honeydew, dark grapes, avocado, coconut, apples, pears, pomegranate, mango, sweet pineapple, plums, raisins, dates. *Strictly avoid: Citrus (except small amounts of lemon and lime), kiwi, banana, sour fruits.*

Cooling or Pitta Pacifying Diet *(cont.)*

Cooking Companions (Oils, Spices, and Sweeteners):
Olive oil (extra virgin, cold pressed, organic) is best. Ghee in small quantities can also be used. Coriander, anise, fennel, cardamom, turmeric, cilantro, parsley, rosemary, basil, small quantities of salt (sea salt or rock salt). Use date sugar, whole cane or turbinado sugar in small quantities only.
Strictly avoid: chilies, hot peppers, cayenne, asafoetida (hing), garlic, ginger powder, cinnamon, refined sugar.

Beverages: Pomegranate juice, lime water, sweet lassi, grape juice, mango juice, coconut-pineapple juice, licorice tea, fennel tea, mint tea.

Special Foods: Lemon and lime are citrus fruit that can be used in cooking that have a special cooling property in spite of their sourness. Cilantro and its seed (coriander) are particularly good for pitta. Pomegranate juice can be taken (you may dilute 50:50 with water for taste) and is particularly good for pitta.

Maximize Your Knowledge

Dispersing/Reducing or Kapha Pacifying Diet

General Principle: Take foods that are light, dry, and well-spiced. Favor tastes that are pungent, bitter, and astringent. Take less food and enjoy it more.

Grains: Barley (the best), millet, buckwheat, rye, oats, quinoa, couscous. *(Rice or pasta: Limit to 1-2 times per week.)*

High-Protein Foods: All beans and peas. Small portions of sunflower, sesame, pumpkin seeds. For non-vegetarians: chicken (only if strong cravings for meat). *Strictly avoid: dairy, processed soy products.*

Vegetables: All vegetables (especially greens) except potatoes, beets, sweet potato.

Fruits: Apples, pears, papaya, guava, pomegranate, cranberry, figs (soaked). *Strictly avoid: banana, avocado, coconut, citrus, sour fruits.*

Dispersing/Reducing or Kapha Pacifying Diet *(cont.)*

Cooking Companions (Oils, Spices, and Sweeteners): Sesame, mustard, or olive oil (extra virgin, cold pressed, organic). Minimal quantity of any oil (as little as possible). All spices except salt. Particularly good: ginger, black pepper, mustard seeds, oregano, sage, thyme, mint, basil, turmeric, cinnamon, cloves. Use only very small amounts of salt while cooking, and do not add salt at meal. Use small amounts of honey for sweetener, but don't cook with it. Otherwise, use turbinado sugar in small quantities only. *Strictly avoid: butter, ghee.*

Beverages: Digestive lassi, ginger tea, fruit juice (from any of the fruits listed above).

Special Foods: Ginger root, daikon radish, digestive lassi.

Maximize Your Knowledge

Tonification or Vata Pacifying Diet

General Principle: Take foods that are heavy, moist, oily, and strengthening (full of prana or life force). Avoid light, dry, raw, crispy foods. Favor more dairy and nuts in the diet. Favor sweet, sour, and salty tastes.

Grains: Quinoa, bulgur wheat, rice (white basmati, Texmati, or jasmine), couscous, pasta (eggless), flat bread made without yeast or baking soda such as chapatis or tortillas.

High-Protein Foods: Moong bean (split or whole), red lentils, green lentils, brown lentils, tofu, pumpkin seeds, almonds (blanched is best). For nonvegetarians: chicken, turkey, fish, eggs. *Strictly avoid: large beans such as pinto beans, kidney beans, black beans, chickpeas.*

Tonification or Vata Pacifying Diet (cont.)

Vegetables: Asparagus, zucchini, fennel, carrot, tomato, artichokes, cucumber, yellow squash, okra, baby eggplant, spinach, red or green chard, snow peas, peas, winter squashes, sweet potato. *Strictly avoid: salads, raw vegetables (except freshly juiced), potatoes, cauliflower, brussels sprouts.*

Fruits: Grapes, plums, cherries, kiwi, peach, apricot, mango, papaya, pineapple, berries, oranges, grapefruit, dates. Also raisins, figs, prunes (soaked overnight or until soft). *Strictly avoid: raw apples, bananas, raw pears.*

Cooking Companions (Oils, Spices, and Sweeteners): Olive oil (extra virgin, cold pressed, organic), ghee. Cumin, ginger, mustard seeds, celery seeds, fenugreek, asafoetida (hing), cinnamon, cardamom, cloves, anise, fennel, black pepper, salt. Use date sugar, whole cane or turbinado sugar in small quantities only. *Strictly avoid: chilies, hot peppers, cayenne, garlic powder.*

Beverages: Digestive lassi, ginger tea, fennel tea, fruit juice (from any of the fruits listed above).

Special Foods: Ghee (1/2 tsp can be taken with the first bite of lunch and dinner). Milk (organic, nonhomogenized is best — be sure to boil and take while warm — best taken before bedtime with 1 tsp ghee and a pinch of cardamom).

> ## *Maximize Your Knowledge*
>
> **Moisturizing or Light Vata Diet**
>
> **General Principle:** The Moisturizing or Light Vata Diet is the same as the Tonification or Vata Pacifying Diet, except that only moderate amounts of oils are taken, and milk and dairy products are not whole milk, rather 1% or 2%. Very heavy foods (like meat or avocadoes) are avoided.

These diets are to be followed for several months (two to four) in order to have the desired impact on rebalancing the physiology. After that process is complete, the next step is rejuvenation. For that process, your ultimate diet is recommended. What is your ultimate diet? We need to cover two more principles to reach the ultimate answer.

* 8 *

Intuitive Eating

Everyone has a doctor in him; I just need to help him in his work.
— Hippocrates

I started this book by explaining that Enlightened
Nutrition is about you. Your experiences can serve as a
guide to the principles behind your ultimate diet if you
put your attention on them. That "if " is important. I
emphasized that of all the principles in the book,
awareness holds the key. Awareness is *the* most
important element in your ultimate diet. Without
awareness, you cannot learn from your experience.
With it, the principles become self-evident. Awareness
can be guided through certain experiences. It can also
be expanded through meditation. The practice of

meditation is key to the rapid development of awareness that makes many of these principles easy to assimilate. Awareness is key to the experiences in this book and forms the basis of its principles.

I have yet to present your ultimate diet. The principles described so far give much of its basis—so much so, that it is time to review what I have presented thus far:

Principle #1: Food conveys life energy.
Implications: Do not take lifeless food. Avoid dead and dumb (unintelligent) foods. Fresh vegetarian food that is close to the source and organic without preservatives or artificial flavors is best.

Principle #2: Food conveys emotion and consciousness.
Implications: The thoughts and emotions of the cook are an important aspect of nutrition. Who prepares your food, the care they put into that preparation, and their relationship with you is important. Home-cooked food, prepared by a loving and spiritual cook is best.

Principle #3: Food immediately starts re-creating the body.
Implications: Optimizing digestion is as important as optimizing the type of food you eat. Digestion can be improved.

Principle #4: When digestion is incomplete, toxins are formed that block metabolism.
Implications: Regular purification of the body is important. Avoiding foods and habits that block digestion is key.

Principle #5: The body constantly seeks to maintain balance.

Implications: Diet can be used to bring about balance and regain health. Food is medicine.

These principles and their implications start to form a broader picture of diet. Diet involves more than just what food is put in the mouth. It incorporates the process of eating, the eater, and the food. The first chapters focused on food. Next, the focus shifted to the process of eating. This chapter focuses more on the eater.

Each individual is unique. Ultimately, no one can prescribe the perfect diet for someone else. Bodies come in different sizes and shapes. They have difference metabolisms. They develop at different rates. They change with time and have different states of balance or imbalance on any given day. Subjecting someone to a diet with exactly so many calories, so much protein and so much fat denies these differences. How could anyone ever know the exact number of calories someone else's body will need in one day? How can one guarantee that the amount of protein or fat is too much by a gram or two? Surely, that extra gram or two will turn into *ama*. A gram or two may not seem like much. But day after day, what would be the effects of creating a gram or two of *ama*?

This is the problem with rule-based diets. That is why the ultimate diet is not a set of rules. It is a set of principles. For digestion to be perfect and *ama* to be avoided, diet must be individualized. Even the best psychic would have difficulty tailoring a diet that is perfect for someone else for the long run.

Each of us has been given our own intuitive abilities. Each of us has within an elaborate feedback mechanism, more sophisticated than the most advanced computer. Each of us has the means to know exactly what we need to eat ... and when. Unfortunately, with all the rules and regulations that are attached to diet, this wondrous system is too easily ignored. We just don't listen. And listening is key to the ultimate diet.

Listening means paying attention to what your gut is saying. It means attending to the sensations you have before you eat, when you are eating, and after you eat. It means having your awareness attuned to your body. When this is the state of mind, then amazing information is available to you. This next experiment gives some hint at what is possible.

Experiment #7

The Gut Feeling Experience

This exercise involves developing your awareness of the sensations in the body. In order to heighten these sensations, you will cut back drastically on food intake for less than one day. The objective is to become aware of the messages the body is giving you.

Required Materials:
  None.

Method:
- For breakfast, take only 1/2 your normal amount of food.
- For lunch, take only 1/4 your normal amount of food.
- Do not skip meals.
- Do not snack between meals.
- Do not dramatically increase your fluid intake.
- If you are not hungry by dinnertime, take only 1/4 the amount of your normal dinner.

Record your experience of hunger during the day by paying particular attention to:

- The sensation of hunger in your gut.
- The type of food you would like to consume.
- The types of taste you would like to take while you are hungry.
- How the hunger changes when you start to eat meals.
- What food tastes you would like to experience at the beginning of the meal, during the middle of the meal, and at the end of the meal.

For this experiment, it is very important to record your impressions. After you have recorded your experiences, you can take a little more for dinner. If hunger did not come until after dinner, then you can take some warm milk or a date shake (for recipe see page 131) to quell the hunger, *after* you have recorded your impressions.

Questions for you to ponder:

1. If you craved a particular taste, why might that be? Would any taste have satisfied?

2. Was the desire to fill the stomach with anything, or was the it for something in particular?

3. If the desire was for something in particular, was this desire coming from the mind or from the gut?

4. Why might the desire change as you start to eat? If it did change, what did it change to?

5. Could you distinguish between what the mind imagined as food and what the gut desired?

That last question refers to what many people describeas "having a gut feeling." We call it that when we are using our intuition. Our minds can conjure up any craving. Our "gut" guides us on the level of feeling to the correct conclusion. Listen to some of the experiences of my patients as they learned about making this distinction.

"I started craving pasta. Now I am a big chocolate fan. I usually think I could live on chocolate, and I anticipated that I would crave this constantly. I was surprised to find myself craving noodles with a little bit of salt and butter. It seems that my body knew it needed to take on some carbs ..."
— Angela B., Graphics Design Artist

"I did not notice very much, except that I was hungry. It was a different kind of hunger, though. It became very intense, and I knew that I wanted something substantial. It was not a desire for desserts or sweets or anything like that. If anything, a submarine

sandwich would have done the trick."
— *Joseph J., Minister*

"At the first full meal I took, I started out with some bread. Then my body seemed to be craving salad. Then it seemed to want some liquid. Then it changed again and it wanted something starchy. Eventually, I was full, but very, very satisfied. The hunger seemed to heighten the experience of each taste, and I enjoyed the contrasts."
— *Margaret P., Housewife*

"All I could think about in the afternoon was cheesecake. I kept entertaining the idea of what kind of cheesecake I might have after the experiment was over. But then, as dinner approached, I noticed that I stopped thinking about it so much. My hunger was deep in the pit of my stomach, and I decided to have some stir-fried tofu and veggies. It seemed to be very much what my body wanted. My mind stopped thinking entirely about cheesecake. I just had an apple for dessert."
— *Paul S., Computer Programmer*

"It was very clear to me what my body was asking for. That feeling deep in the stomach was so clear to me. It was as if it was talking to me, telling me what to eat next. First, one taste, then the next. First, one texture, then the next. I noticed I ate more slowly, and I also ate less than usual, but was completely satisfied."
— *Jenny B., Yoga Instructor*

Some people know precisely what the body is craving. Others need to develop this awareness. Regardless, most make the distinction between what foods the mind is thinking about and what the body is asking for. Nine times out of 10, people do not go for junk food after restricting their diet for a short time. Most do not binge on chocolate.

Learning to distinguish between what foods the mind might find pleasing or entertaining and what the gut is calling out for is paramount to intuitive eating. The experience of true hunger can heighten this distinction. Intuitive eating calls for listening to the body and not getting involved in the habits and cravings of the mind. This is a constant process. It does occur for a few seconds before you reach into the refrigerator. Constant awareness is a part of conscious eating. It is the key to detecting a change in what the body is requiring in this instant. When it is refined, each bite is followed by a shift in sensation and a reassessment of what the body is calling out for. Is something sour needed now? Is something heavy needed next? Is something crunchy needed now? Is something sweet needed next? This constant attending to the signals of the body guides the process of eating. It assures the development of the most important feedback system in the body. It is the key to healthful eating.

Our society has such difficulty with food and eating that diets become rules for suppressing our desires. Desire is the means through which the body expresses its needs. Desiring a salty taste or a sweet taste or a bitter taste is the body's communication method. Ignoring and suppressing desire damages this feedback system and makes one less aware. It often results in mental tension. This produces cravings. Cravings can be out of a sense of deprivation, or they can result from specific imbalances. Mental cravings distract you from the messages of the body. The gut feeling you intuitively have is overridden by the mind's insistence on a specific sensation. Mental cravings of a persistent nature sometimes have meaning. They sometimes relate to an imbalance in the physiology. Below is a list of the meanings of some cravings.

THE INSIDE SCOOP

The Meaning of Cravings

Cravings are sometimes the result of imbalances in the physiology or the diet. When they are present, they can give a clue as to what changes are needed in the diet. Below are some common cravings and their potential implications.

CRAVING FOR SWEETS AFTER A MEAL IN NONOBESE PERSON: *Can mean protein deficiency; diet is not rich enough or heavy enough to ground the individual.*

CRAVING FOR SALT: *Can be sluggish digestion. Digestion needs to be sharpened. Activity level is too high and digestion is being damaged by overdoing.*

CRAVING FOR HOT SPICY FOODS: *Can be weak digestion, particularly from lack of exercise and physical activity.*

CRAVING FOR SOUR: *Can be from the buildup of ama. Ama needs to be cut through and dissolved for digestion to work right.*

CRAVING FOR BITTER *(such as coffee or dark chocolate): Can be lack of bitter in the diet (not enough greens and vegetables).*

Learning to eat intuitively is the most important skill you can develop in regard to your health. Your intuition is more sophisticated than any computer. It can provide the exact ingredients you need to properly nourish and reconstruct the body. It is in each of us. It only needs to be developed.

Intuition is tied to having that "gut feeling" about something. It is deep in the gut that we experience a more refined feeling about what is right for us. Practice refines it. It promotes it and allows it to expand. Eating intuitively has another advantage over prescribed diets — it is fun. When you satisfy the body's desires (as opposed the mind's cravings), you feel completely fulfilled. You experience complete satisfaction, not a temporary fleeting pause in craving.

Eating intuitively is ultimately the way you can assure that your body is well-nourished. It is part of our distrust of nature, our desire to "conquer the elements" that makes us distrustful of the body's desires. This has caused many generations of parents to impose their ideas about diet and eating on their children.

In order to discover whether children really need such guidance, researchers undertook to study what happens when children are given complete freedom to choose their diet without guidance from the outside. The research project utilized a gymnasium with tables stocked with different diet elements. There was a dessert table, a snack table, a vegetable table, a bread table, etc. The children were brought to the gym for meals and given free reign to eat whatever they wanted in whatever quantity they wanted. Many of the researchers predicted that the children would just eat sweet snacks and desserts and would never choose a balanced diet. What they found was that those children who had been deprived of having sweets binged for a few days on desserts, but by the end of a week, almost all of the children were eating a balanced diet. By the end of two weeks, they all were taking foods from every food group. Without supervision, the children naturally gravitated to a healthful diet.

This study points out the intelligence that is innate in the body. It demonstrates the role desire can play in modifying diet for health. Desire is not the enemy—not listening to the body is. This leads us to our sixth principle:

Principle #6: Desire is the body's mechanism for communicating its needs.

Awareness of this communication and refinement to pinpoint the exact message can be developed. This again points to the importance of consciousness and the development of greater awareness through meditation. As consciousness develops, so does intuition. Refinement of intuition can be enhanced to the point that the need for specific foods in the diet can be ascertained. The key here is practice. Practice referring to yourself for guidance. Practice paying attention as you eat to the desires of the body. Practice distinguishing the fascination of the mind for some taste from the desire of the body.

Some help may be in order for those who struggle constantly with sugar cravings. Sugar cravings are particularly hard for some people to sort out. As mentioned above, in a thin person who is taking a restrictive diet, this can be the body's cry for more nourishment. Higher protein intake and richer, more soothing foods may be indicated. For other individuals, taking dessert or ingesting sugar-laden drinks may be a mental habit. Breaking that habit can be difficult, particularly in people struggling with weight issues. To break this habit by sheer willpower is sometimes difficult. The ancient knowledge of herbs and herbal combinations are sometimes used to help. Most herbal weight-loss products act as stimulants, unfortunately. They whip an already tired horse resulting in side effects of heart arrhythmias and nausea. The ancient physicians knew better than to take this route. They addressed the problem on another level — on the level of emotion and intuition.

Maintaining normal weight is not a matter of ingesting a diet pill. That is why studies found that meditators' weight tended to normalize soon after they began the practice of meditation. In order for the body's feedback system to do its job, it is important to pay attention to how you eat. Likewise, it is important to break some old habits and conditioning.

THE INSIDE SCOOP

The Spiritually Clean Plate Club

The current concept is that if you leave food on your plate, you are being wasteful. This mentality led to the "clean plate club," where you were rewarded for finishing every bite of food on your plate. This concept comes from an attitude of insufficiency. While it materially honors the food and its value, it is not so pure from the spiritual viewpoint.

The ancient seers knew that eating when you were already full would create ama. Not only would it be a waste of food, it would help to destroy the eater's health. In that sense, eating food because it is placed on the plate is doubly wasted. It honors neither the food nor the eater.

With this knowledge, it would be best to adopt a different attitude and a different practice. I call this the Spiritually Clean Plate Club because it honors Nature and the eater at the same time. It is the opposite of the materially clean plate club. And it encourages you to tune into the body to determine when you are full. It works as follows:

1) Never eat all the food on your plate.
2) Always leave a portion that is going to be given back to Nature as thanks for nourishing and supporting your life.
3) Always check to see when you are getting full — stop eating at 75% - 80% full.
4) If possible, utilize that portion left on the plate for composting and nourishing the soil near your home.

This practice encourages respect for Nature, respect for you, and it helps you to develop greater awareness of the body and when it is full.

Two other caveats are important in developing intuitive eating. The first is eating slowly. Just shoveling in food after you have intuited what your body needs will assure you miss any necessary changes that occur as the body starts to metabolize things. As you chew, the taste of food changes. Chewing thoroughly is important for digestion. It slows the process so that you can attend to the taste. Too often people eat and don't experience the food. They walk away hungry. Eating slowly and enjoying the taste of the food is key.

The other important point is to have available all six tastes at a meal. As the body shifts and needs a different taste, it helps to have this available on the table to meet the body's need. Too often bitter and astringent tastes are missing from the typical diet. In order to help supply this I offer a recipe for Swiss chard. The chard has a wonderful bitterness to it. Placing lemon juice on it at the end gives it an astringency that delights the palate and makes the mouth want to pucker. This recipe can easily be varied with other greens that also supply the much-needed bitter taste in the diet.

*** See Recipe for Health - Swiss Chard in Appendix II ***

* 9 *

Metabolizing The Universe

You are what you eat.
—Anonymous

What we eat, we become. Food and its qualities form our bodies and determine their qualities. What comes in from the external environment becomes the internal environment. It is a fascinating process. But it is only part of the story. We know that the point of life is not to eat. We do not live to eat. We eat to live. Ultimately diet supports the ability of the brain to experience love, happiness, and fulfillment. Diet is central to the maintenance of health. But it is also essential to our experience. The quality of our experience is intimately dependent on diet. Why is this? How can diet be so important?

The process of incorporating the external into the internal goes on in more ways than one. Just as blood, muscle, and bone are constantly being rejuvenated and reconstructed, so too is the brain. And just as the quality of muscle tissue created is dependent on the quality of the food taken, so too is the quality of experience dependent on the brain's diet. Brain cells don't generally die off and regenerate the way blood cells do. For this reason, many scientists used to think the brain was fairly static and unchanging. Today we know it is not.

First, each brain cell has its own housekeeping chores. The molecules that make up the average brain cell are replaced and recycled. They are reconstructed routinely just as other cells are recreated. What is more important, brain cells are modified. When an area of the brain is used, the connections between the cells are strengthened. The brain cells send out little arms (dendrites) that interface with surrounding cells. The more an area of the brain is used, the greater the number of dendrites. When an area of the brain is not used, the number of connections decrease. This amazing capability of the brain is what is referred to as "neural plasticity." This allows a stroke victim, for example, to recover functions that were wiped out initially by the stroke. Other parts of the brain start to take over the functions of the dead tissue and form new connections. In some cases, this is sufficient for a full recovery of function.

What this means is that whatever you take in from the environment gets incorporated into the brain. If you start playing tennis with your left hand, the right motor cortex of the brain changes its connections. If you start listening to Mozart five hours a day, the auditory center in the brain is stimulated, and new connections are created. (By the way, these connections are different from those formed by rock 'n' roll). If you watch television three hours a day, that also changes the brain connections. Whatever we experience alters the physical functioning and aspect of the brain.

The implication is that diet is much more than food. In fact, food is only a small part of diet. The experience of eating is an important part of diet. But experience itself is diet. This broader definition of diet can be stated as follows:

Diet is anything that is taken in by the brain, whether it is through the senses, the mind, or the mouth.

Whatever we experience, we metabolize, and it becomes part of who we are. Our ability to digest experience allows us to incorporate it into the physical body. What we eat becomes us. Likewise, what we see, we become. Each experience affects us and how the brain functions. Our next experiment will demonstrate some of this. For most people, this will have to be a thought experiment, as it involves a sophisticated set-up with colored lights in a darkened room. It is based on some research on color done in the 1960s.

Experiment #8

The Color Experience

Method: This experiment is done is a darkened room with focused spotlights. The lights are focused on a dinner table where various items are placed, such as a cup of tea, a salad, vegetable soup, and a pasta main dish. Each dish is separated from the other so that each is lit by a single spotlight. Each spotlight has a different color. The color scheme is designed to create the following effects:

- The tea is blood red

- The soup is bright yellow-green

- The pasta is violet, bordering on black

- The salad is bright red

If you are unable to arrange such an experiment, just picture in your mind how you would feel sitting down to eat at this table. Record your impressions.

The original experiment involved meat-eaters, and the steak was made to look bright green. Rather than giving you feedback from our patients this time, I will give you some of the results of the original experiment.

Almost without exception, the experimental subjects ate less than they usually did. Many rated the meal poor-tasting, even though it was the exact same meal they had rated highly the day before. Some people could not eat at all. Some actually became nauseated at the sight of the food. Just this one environmental change had a profound impact on digestion and on experience. Why?

THE SCIENCE BEHIND THE SAGES

THE EFFECT OF COLOR ON FOOD PERCEPTION

Color is a powerful visual cue in conferring meaning to food: The unexpected pairing of a given food with a novel color may render the food unpalatable. The following anecdote illustrates this point:

" ... prepared a buffet of goods for a dinner with scientific colleagues of the Flavor Group of the Society of Chemistry and Industry in London. Many of the foods were inappropriately colored, and during the dinner several individuals complained about the off-flavor of many of the foods served. Several of the individuals reported feeling ill after eating some of the foods, despite the fact that only the color was varied. The rest of the food was perfectly wholesome, with the requisite taste, smell, and texture."

In the 1990s, PepsiCo Inc. launched "Crystal Pepsi." Apart from its clear color, Crystal Pepsi was identical to regular Pepsi in all respects. Unfortunately, the PepsiCo failed to consider the possibility of a food color/flavor interaction. To cola drinkers, "clearness" conveys "noncola" flavor expectations. Consequently, cola drinkers trying Crystal Pepsi for the first time were bowled over by its full flavor.

In a taste-test experiment manipulating food color and label information, 389 undergraduates at a public university (53% male and 47% female; 79% between 18 and 21 years of age) were asked to evaluate a successful brand of powdered fruit drink. Results from this study indicated that food color affected the consumer's ability to correctly identify flavor and to form distinct flavor profiles and preferences. Food color was the most dominant source of flavor information, including written labeling and actual drink taste.

Mind, emotion, and digestion are intimately linked. What we feel with our gut is intimately related to what biochemicals are produced in the brain. In fact, both brain cells and cells in the gut share receptors for the same hormone-like substances (neuropeptides). Mind and emotion nurture and nourish the brain, just as food nourishes the blood. It works the other way also. When the mind is overwhelmed with external stimuli, the brain produces biochemical messengers that affect the gut. They can shut down digestion, or they can make one nauseated at the sight of food — even the best food. This leads us to the most important principle reflecting this broader definition of diet:

Principle #7: Diet is everything taken in through experience. Therefore, what we see, we become.

In order to create a perfect body, we need to be taking in perfection on the level of experience. In order to create a peaceful, loving mind, we need to be experiencing a state of peace and love. In order to create a body full of energy, we need to be contacting and experiencing a source of infinite energy. This may sound mystical, but I am not responsible for the way the body works. It may also sound impossible. I assure you it is not.

THE SCIENCE BEHIND THE SAGES

YOUR GUT HAS A MIND OF ITS OWN

"Indigestion is the base of all physical diseases, the condition from which all other disease conditions arise. In a sense, indigestion, the inability of an individual to digest any physical, mental, or emotional input, is the sole disease of a living being. It usually begins in the mind as an 'offense against wisdom' and is projected from the mind into the physical body." [***Cite: Svoda (1998), "Prakriti" p. 115]

Our nervous system (vata) controls the digestive force (kapha and pitta) in our stomach and intestines. If our nervous system is not working properly, it will likely throw our digestive ability off-balance. This, in turn, may further negatively impact our nervous system thereby creating a vicious cycle of disorder.

This ancient knowledge has only recently been articulated in Western medicine. In his book, "The Second Brain," the renowned scientist Michael Gershon, M.D., recounts 30 years of research that went into understanding the functioning of the human digestive system. He is touted to be the "father of neurogastroenterology" because his work elucidated the intimate relationship between the nervous and digestive systems. In the late 1960s he reported on the existence of a neurotransmitter that both worked on and was produced by cells of the intestines: serotonin.

Previously, this neurotransmitter was relegated to functioning *solely* in the brain. The implications of this finding were radical—could the gut have a mind of its own? Gershon explains:

THE SCIENCE BEHIND THE SAGES (cont.)

"The enteric nervous system is thus an independent site of neural integration and processing. This is what makes it the second brain. The enteric nervous system may never compose syllogisms, write poetry, or engage in Socratic dialogue, but it is a brain nevertheless. It runs its organ, the gut; and if push comes to shove (as it does in the millions of people who have had their vagus nerves surgically interrupted), it can do that all by itself."

The radical concept presented by Gershon is that the "second brain" in the gut may actually have a significant impact on, if not dominion over, the brain in our skull:

"When the enteric nervous system runs the bowel well, there is bliss in the body. When the enteric nervous system fails and the gut acts badly, syllogisms, poetry, and Socratic dialogue all seem to fade into nothingness."
[***Cite: Gershon (1998), p. 17.]

Functional bowel diseases such as irritable bowel syndrome and leaky gut syndrome are still generally considered to originate in the mind (i.e., psychosomatic). Perhaps they will soon be considered to originate in the gut itself—a result of poor digestion, of "offenses against wisdom." Subsequently, treatment for such diseases will focus on what we put into our body (purification of the mind and body), the functioning of the gut (the condition of our digestive fire and balance of the doshas), as well as the state of the individual (level of consciousness).

Doesn't the evidence for the existence of TWO separate-but-equal brains validate the point that we "digest" everything in our universe, everything that we take in through our senses?

Throughout this book, I have emphasized the importance of consciousness and its development. The development of greater awareness is key to better health and to proper diet. But the development of higher consciousness is the key to creating optimal health and fulfilling one's full potential.

It works in a reciprocal fashion. Just as in the color experiment, the mind's experience influences appetite, which in turn influences digestion. Indigestion influences the mind. Whatever we experience repeatedly makes a deeper connection in the brain. Our "diet" from the environment re-creates us in its reflection. Therefore, in order to create the highest level in both body and mind, the highest experience must be cultivated. This can only be done through meditation. What does the mind metabolize in meditation?

Meditation allows the mind to settle and go to the source of thought. Scientists have found that the brain is capable of operating on the level of quantum mechanics. Put succinctly, all matter arises out of an underlying field. This field is the home of all the fundamental forces in creation. It is called the unified field, because it is where the four fundamental forces in physics are unified and act as one. Energy does not arise out of this field in a continual gradient of strength. It jumps out of the field to a level. This is the so-called quantum leap. The smallest amount of light energy that can arise from this field is the photon. It is one quanta of light. Scientists have found that in a completely darkened room the human eye can perceive a single photon of green light. For this to be possible, the retina of the eye has to react to this, and then the nervous system has to amplify this and create a perception. This proves that the nervous system is sensitive down to the level of the quantum field. It is not far-fetched then to suppose that thought is taking place on this subtle level of energy. When one "goes beyond thought" or transcends thought in meditation, then one contacts the underlying unified field.

The unified field is the field out of which all creation arises. When you experience and metabolize the unified field, you are literally metabolizing the entire universe. While metabolizing something that huge may sound like it would cause heartburn, it does not. The experience is one of peace, because the unified field is the resting point out of which creation comes. The unified field is a field of tremendous energy. It is a field of tremendous potentiality. Its experience is one of pure silence and peace that re-energizes the body. Repeated experience of the unified field allows the brain to be cultured to experience the Ultimate Reality. Experiencing and knowing the totality of life is the true purpose of diet. Experiencing the Ultimate Reality is really what the human frame was designed for. The ultimate diet is created to hasten the development of the ability to know the Ultimate Reality. It allows you to fulfill your potential for optimal health and optimal functioning on all levels — mental, emotional, spiritual, and physical.

Maximize Your Knowledge

What You See You Become

- In order to gain the most from this principle of "what you see you become" consider the following:

- Avoid violence in television, in news, in novels, and food (no meat).

- Favor uplifting diet and uplifting inputs such as fine art, classical music, uplifting novels.

- Go for a week without TV, videos, movies, etc. and see how you feel. Remember: Everything that affects your mind alters your brain. The more you repeat an experience, the more that experience and those connections get fixed in the brain.

* 10 *

The Ultimate Diet
for
The Ultimate Reality

Knowledge is structured in consciousness.
— Maharishi Mahesh Yogi

Whether you are a spiritual seeker or just interested in optimizing your health, the principles of Enlightened Nutrition will help you to attain your own ultimate diet. The ultimate diet is not a prescription for so many calories or for 40 or 60 grams of protein. The ultimate diet is a very personal thing. The more we become aware of ourselves and gain the ability to discriminate mental craving from gut desire, the more effective we will be in attaining our personal ultimate potential. The more in tune with our desire, the more we will come to know "intelligent" desires from mental habits.

After you have done one to three weeks of the purification diet and two to four months of rebalancing, you are ready for unlocking your ultimate diet. There are several keys to unlock your personal ultimate potential. Using a key is not the only way to get through a door — it is simply the easiest:

- The key to the ultimate diet is awareness.

- The key to developing awareness is meditation.

- The key to developing meditation is an effective teacher. (See Appendix III for recommendations.)

Short of developing that ultimate awareness, I can help you to understand some of the qualities and characteristics of your ultimate diet. I have not yet presented a formal definition of the ultimate diet, because I did not want you to get bound by someone else's rules. I have tried to give you some experiences throughout the book to help you to understand the principles that guide the healthiest diet. Now I will present our definition:

The ultimate diet is pure organic vegetarian food that is fresh and freshly prepared by a spiritual and loving cook according to the balance needed by the body, satisfying the intuitive desires of the body, and creating wholeness on all levels.

The ultimate diet conveys the life force and liveliness needed by the body. It provides the appropriate qualities in food needed to balance the body. It satisfies deeply. It gives the body exactly what is needed at the moment. It helps you to avoid creating *ama* and keeps digestion proper. It allows you to metabolize food completely into healthy tissue. It nourishes the mind and emotions. Finally and most important, it creates the health you need to fulfill your total potential. That potential extends beyond wellness to the highest of intellectual and spiritual pursuits.

What does the ultimate diet look like? It is a light diet that emphasizes whole grains and legumes. It emphasizes fresh vegetables and fruits. It utilizes fresh dairy products, not aged ones. It is a simple diet. It is very close to the purification diet I described earlier. It incorporates more liberal use of milk and clarified butter (ghee) than did the purification diet. It relies on homemade foods. It is inexpensive. If breakfast is taken, it is usually a cooked grain with or without milk. Lunch is usually a grain with a legume, at least two vegetables, and sometimes lassi. Sometimes pasta is taken instead of grains. Sometimes a fresh cheese (paneer) is taken. But simple foods, freshly prepared, are its essence. Dinner is often smaller than lunch. For those needing more substance to balance their light physique, dinner can be almost a repeat of lunch. For those who need to balance a heavier physique, dinner can be a repeat of breakfast. This is just a general description for the simple reason that the ultimate diet is an individual thing. The principles I have presented in this book are its essence.

The ultimate diet is designed to optimize health. It is designed to be light enough to allow one to use the body's energies for pursuits other than digestion. If the diet is too heavy, it can interfere with the development of greater awareness and greater effectiveness in activity.

Often there are questions about some of the quirks of the diet. Here are common questions I am asked by my patients and how I answer them:

Why the emphasis on vegetarian diet?

Five reasons:

1) Research has shown that it is healthier.
2) Meat is dead food unless you slaughter the animal yourself. It creates dullness in the awareness and *ama* in the body.
3) Meat is extremely hard to digest. It is like trying to digest your own body — it is hard for the digestion to sort out what's what.
4) Cooking meat creates acrylamide — a carcinogen.
5) Meat disturbs the normal bacteria in the colon causing them to produce carcinogenic substances.

Why is milk and dairy considered okay, then?

Milk has a different energy. It is not dead. In fact, in terms of energy, it is one of the purest foods available. Almost all other foods involve loss of life in some form. The plant dies or the seed never sprouts. Milk is the one food that is given freely to nourish and to nurture other beings. Almost all difficulty people have tolerating milk comes from weak digestion (and from not knowing how to prepare it). Milk should be boiled first and taken with spices and not other foods, except grains. For those with very weak digestion it can be taken diluted 50:50 with water. The best spices to use with it are cardamom, cinnamon, and fresh ginger.

Why use clarified butter (ghee)? Isn't all that cholesterol bad for you?

The brain is a very fatty tissue. It has an extremely high cholesterol content. Trying to avoid all cholesterol in the diet is not useful for you if you are trying to restructure how the brain functions (to increase your awareness). Ghee can be overdone, but in moderation it is not harmful. It has very interesting properties as an oil. It is cooling in nature, whereas most oils are heating. It contains very short chain fatty acids (carbon links) that give cells greater fluidity which enables them to be incorporated into cell walls.

Why no onions and garlic?

Some people notice that highly spiritual people on the ultimate diet avoid garlic and onions. These can disturb the mind in very sensitive people. Garlic can dull the mind in some people. Onions can be very stimulating and cause mental distraction. This is not a hard and fast rule. As pointed out before, the key is to become aware and intuit whether these need to be avoided.

Why the emphasis on the consciousness of the cook? How important is this?

We are more than biochemicals. The most important aspects of human life are nonphysical. Food conveys the qualities of the cook to the eater. It can be very important. Just try home cooking for a week or two, and see how you feel.

If this is the ultimate diet, why do so many people seem to be healthy without it?

Our definition of "healthy" is set too low. The human body was designed to live much longer than 70 or 80 years. Because of poor dietary habits, it is just accepted that the body starts wearing out in the 70's. If people knew that their diet was robbing them of 30 or 40 years of life, they might reconsider what is healthy.

How can anyone find the time to do all this?

Some hints have been given along the way as to how to make this approach to diet practical by utilizing modern conveniences — a rice cooker, a crockpot, an oven that has a timer, thermos-meals, etc. What I have found, though, is the key to finding the time is twofold:

1) Make it a priority.

2) Make it enjoyable.

If you start enjoying your food twice as much as before, it will be easy to spend more time on it. In addition, if you understand that a huge part of the illnesses seen today are related to diet, then you will realize that every minute you invest is well worth it. Who among us can afford to sacrifice their health to cram more activity into their day?

Do I have to become a spiritual person to take advantage of the ultimate diet?

If you mean a reverent person who engages in religious rituals and practices, then no. Life is spiritual, regardless of whether you recognize it or engage in formal religions. Taking a moment before eating to give thanks to Nature has a practical purpose of preparing one's awareness to focus on the food and to digest it well. While you do not have to be spiritual to take advantage of the ultimate diet, over time, the diet will allow your connection with Nature to grow. In that sense, you will become more spiritual from the diet, not the other way around.

The purpose of the ultimate diet is to create optimal health. Health comes from the old English *hale,* meaning to make whole. It means reconnecting with the source of wholeness that supports all of life. It requires reconnecting with the wholeness that underlies all of Nature. This reconnecting is done in part through honoring and respecting Nature. It involves honoring our individual natures and desires. It is further promoted through metabolizing lively and intelligent aspects of Nature. It is ultimately promoted through transcending the mind and metabolizing the entire universe.

Most of the problems of health and disease relate to diet and to the lack of being in tune with Nature and with one's true nature. The ultimate diet will allow you to become in tune with Nature once again and thereby regain health. If the ultimate diet and the American diet were one and the same, health care would be transformed, the aggressive trends in society would be diminished, and the world would be transformed.

This book began with the statement that it is about your experience. If your experience is not what you want it to be, then I ask you to consider the points in this book. Trust yourself, and use your experience to guide you to greater health. In doing so, you create a better world.

Appendix I

Ayurvedic Food Properties

Ayurvedic Food Properties

Increasing (+) or decreasing (-) or neutral effect (*)

VEGETABLES	V	P	K	QUALITIES
Artichoke	-	-	+	Sweet, Heavy, Cold
Asparagus	-	*	+	Sweet, Heavy
Avocado	-	*	+	Sweet, Oily, Heavy
Bean Sprouts	+	-	-	Sweet, Bitter, Light
Beets	-	-	+	Sweet, Astringent, Heavy
Beet Greens	+	-	-	Sweet, Bitter, Astringent
Broccoli	+	-	-	Sweet, Astringent, Bitter
Brussels Sprouts	+	-	-	Sweet, Salty, Bitter, Astringent
Cabbage	+	-	-	Sweet, Bitter, Astringent
Carrots	*	-	-	Sweet, Bitter
Cauliflower	+	-	*	Sweet, Salty, Astringent,
Celery	+	-	-	Astringent, Light
Cucumbers	-	-	+	Sweet, Cold, Heavy
Eggplant	+	-	-	Sweet, Light, Astringent
Green Beans	-	*	-	Sweet
Lettuce	+	-	-	Sweet, Bitter, Astringent, Light
Peas	+	*	-	Sweet, Astringent, Light
Pepper (sweet)	-	*	+	Sweet, Sharp
Peppers (hot)	+	+	-	Pungent, Astringent
Potato	+	-	+	Sweet, Astringent, Heavy
Radish	-	+	-	Pungent
Spinach	+	*	-	Astringent, Light, Hot
Tomato	-	+	+	Sweet, Sour, Light
Swiss Chard	+	-	-	Bitter
Squash	+	-	-	Sweet, Dry, Heavy
Yam	*	-	+	Sweet, Astringent, Heavy
Zucchini	+	-	-	Sweet, Astringent, Heavy
Zucchini (peeled)	*	-	-	Sweet, Astringent, Cold
GRAINS				
Barley	+	-	-	Sweet, Astringent, Light
Corn	*	+	-	Sweet, Astringent, Hot, Light
Millet	*	*	-	Sweet, Light
Oats	+	-	+	Sweet, Astringent, Heavy
Rice (white)	-	-	+	Sweet, Cold, Light, Oily
Rice (brown)	+	-	+	Rough, Heavy, Sweet, Cold
Rye	-	+	-	Sour, Hot
Wheat	-	-	+	Sweet, Cold, Oily, Heavy

LENTILS AND BEANS				
Moong (Mung) Lentils	+	-	-	Astringent, Light, Cold
Red Lentils	+	-	-	Astringent, Light, Cold
Urad Lentils	-	-	+	Sweet, Astringent, Heavy, Hot
Kidney Beans	+	-	+	Astringent, Dry, Heavy
Pinto Beans	+	-	+	Astringent, Dry, Heavy
Other Beans	+	-	+	Astringent, Dry, Heavy
Tofu and other Soybean Products	*	-	+	Sweet, Heavy, Cold
DAIRY PRODUCTS				
Milk (cow's)	-	-	+	Sweet, Oily, Heavy, Cold
Buttermilk	-	+	+	Sour, Cold, Heavy
Butter	-	-	+	Sweet, Sour, Oily, Soft
Sour Cream	-	+	+	Sour, Cold, Heavy
Yogurt	-	+	+	Sour, Cool, Heavy, Oily
Lassi	-	-	+	Sour, Cool
Panir, Ricotta Cheese	-	-	+	Sweet, Heavy, Oily, Cold
Cottage Cheese	-	*	+	Sweet, Sour, Cold
Semi-hard and Hard Cheese	-	+	+	Sour, Cold, Heavy, Oily
OILS				
Coconut	-	-	+	Sweet, Very Heavy, Oily
Ghee	-	-	+	Sweet, Light, Cold, Oily
Olive	-	-	+	Sweet, Astringent, Oily
Sesame	-	+	+	Sweet, Bitter, Heating, Oily
Sunflower	-	-	+	Sweet, Light, Oily
Safflower	-	+	-	Sweet, Pungent, Heating
SEEDS AND NUTS				
Almonds (blanched)	-	-	+	Sweet, Heavy, Oily
Sesame seeds	-	+	+	Sweet, Bitter, Heavy, Oily
Sunflower (raw)	-	-	+	Sweet, Heavy
Walnuts	+	-	-	Astringent, Bitter
Cashews	-	-	+	Sweet, Heavy
Peanuts	-	+	+	Sweet, Sour, Heavy

FRUITS	V	P	K	QUALITIES
Apples	+	-	*	Sweet, Astringent, Light, Cold
Apples (Stewed)	-	-	*	Sweet, Warm
Apricots	-	*	+	Sweet, Slightly Sour
Banana	-	-	+	Sweet, Heavy, Smooth
Cherries	-	-	+	Sweet, Heavy
Coconut	-	-	+	Sweet, Very Oily, Heavy
Cranberries	-	*	+	Sweet, Sour, Astringent
Currents	-	-	+	Sweet
Dates	-	-	+	Sweet, Heavy
Figs	-	-	+	Sweet, Heavy
Grapes	-	-	+	Sweet, Cold
Grapefruit	-	+	+	Sour, Sharp
Kiwi	-	-	+	Sweet, Cold
Lemon	-	*	+	Sour, Astringent
Lime	-	-	+	Slightly Sour
Mango	-	*	+	Sweet, Sour, Cold
Melons	-	-	+	Sweet, Cold, Heavy
Orange (sweet)	-	*	+	Sweet, Sour
Orange (sour)	-	+	+	Sour, Sharp, Heavy
Peaches	-	-	+	Sweet, Slightly Sour, Heavy
Pears (ripe or dried)	-	-	+	Sweet, Heavy, Cold
Pineapple (fresh)	-	-	+	Sweet, Slightly Sour, Cold
Pomegranate	+	-	-	Astringent, Sweet, Sour
Prunes/Plums	-	-	+	Sweet, Slightly Sour, Heavy
Raisins	-	-	+	Sweet
Raspberries	-	-	+	Sweet, Slightly Bitter
Strawberries	-	*	+	Sweet, Slightly Sour
Watermelon	-	-	+	Sweet, Light, Cold
SWEETENERS				
Honey	+	-	-	Sweet, Astringent, Heavy
Molasses	-	-	+	Sweet, Heavy
Sugars	-	-	+	Sweet, Heavy, Cold
HERBS AND SPICES				
Anise	*	-	-	Sweet, Bitter, Astringent
Asafoetida	-	+	-	Pungent, Astringent
Basil	-	+	-	Pungent
Bay Leaves	*	+	-	Bitter, Astringent
Caraway	-	*	+	Bitter, Astringent
Cardamom	-	-	-	Sweet, Pungent, Cooling
Cayenne	+	+	-	Pungent, Light, Dry
Celery Seed	-	*	-	Pungent, Bitter
Chili Pepper	+	+	-	Pungent, Dry, Hot
Cilantro	*	-	-	Pungent, Astringent, Bitter
Cinnamon	-	*	-	Pungent, Bitter, Sweet

Cloves	-	+	-	Pungent, Bitter, Light
Coriander	*	-	-	Sweet, Astringent, Bitter, Pungent
Cumin	-	+	-	Sweet, Bitter, Pungent, Light
Dill	-	-	*	Bitter, Astringent
Fennel	-	-	*	Sweet, Bitter, Pungent
Fenugreek	-	+	-	Sweet, Bitter, Hot
Garlic	-	+	+	Sour, Pungent, Drying
Ginger	-	+	-	Pungent, Sweet, Light, Cry
Horseradish	+	+	-	Bitter, Light
Lemon Thyme	*	+	-	Pungent
Licorice Root	-	-	-	Sweet, Light
Marjoram	+	+	-	Pungent, Slightly Astringent
Mustard	-	+	-	Pungent, Oily, Sharp, Hot
Nutmeg	+	-	-	Bitter, Sweet, Dry
Oregano	+	+	-	Pungent, Slightly Astringent
Paprika	-	+	-	Sweet, Slightly Pungent
Parsley	-	*	-	Pungent, Astringent, Slightly Bitter
Pepper (black)	-	+	-	Pungent, Dry, Light, Hot
Poppy Seed	-	-	+	Bitter
Rosemary	+	+	-	Astringent, Slightly Bitter, Sharp
Saffron	-	-	-	Sweet, Pungent
Sage	+	+	-	Pungent, Astringent, Bitter
Salt	-	+	+	Pungent, Smooth, Heavy
Sesame Seed	-	+	+	Sweet, Astringent, Bitter
Tarragon	+	+	-	Pungent, Bitter
Thyme	+	+	-	Pungent, Astringent, Slightly Bitter
Turmeric	-	-	-	Bitter, Astringent, Pungent
TEAS				
Black Tea	+	*	-	Astringent, Bitter
Chamomile	-	*	-	Bitter, Astringent
Peppermint	*	-	-	Pungent, Sweet, Sharp
Spearmint	*	-	-	Pungent, Sweet, Astringent, Sharp
Rosehips	-	+	*	Sour, Astringent
Jasmine	*	-	-	Astringent, Bitter, Sweet

Appendix II

Recipes for Health

Basmati Rice

The best way to prepare basmati rice is to first rinse it in water. Place the desired amount in a large bowl, cover with water, and then strain out the water at least three times, checking for small stones. After the rice is thoroughly rinsed, place it in the cooking pot and allow it soak in water for 15 - 30 minutes. This allows each grain to absorb water and thereby stick less to other grains while cooking. Sautéing also helps to prevent sticking. If you do not soak the rice first, cook one part rice to two parts water.

Soaked rice can use less water such as 1 cup of rice to 1¾ cups water. Bring the rice and water to a boil, cover with a secure lid, and reduce to a simmer. Don't lift the lid or stir the rice as it is cooking. The reason is that as the rice is expanding it forms various steam tunnels. If these are interrupted then the rice will not cook evenly, resulting in the bottom being soggy or burned and the top not done.   Allow to cook for 15 - 20 minutes. The rice should not be mushy and stuck together. Each grain should come out firm, separate, and tasty.

To tell if the rice is cooked enough, remove a grain, and squeeze it between the thumb and forefinger. It should completely mash. There should be no hard parts. Do not add cold water to rice that is already cooking. This destroys the cooking process. Salt should not be added until the rice is finished cooking. Most recipes with rice suggest that you add salt at the beginning, but Ayurveda says that the salt actually affects the temperature of the cooking process, and that then affects the digestibility of the rice. Salt can be mixed in after the rice is cooked.

Ghee

Place four sticks sweet (unsalted) organic butter in a pot on low. Once the butter melts, the water contained in the butter will start to boil and make a distinctive sound. Continue boiling on low heat for approximately 20 minutes. Skim the foam off the top. The rest of the milk solids will drop to the bottom of the pan, and the oil will start to crackle with a high-pitched sound and turn golden brown. Do not overcook or else the butter will burn and the oil will turn dark brown and have a burnt odor. Strain the oil through cheesecloth into a clean jar. (**Be careful not to burn yourself, as the oil is quite hot at this point.**)

Ghee does not have to be refrigerated. It will keep fresh on the countertop for up to a month.

Ginger Chutney

Use: Use as a spice on one's food occasionally,
particularly when the appetite is dull.

Why:
1) Aids digestion and enkindles *jatharagni* (the main
   digestive fire in the stomach)
2) Has post-digestive effect that is cooling, even
   though initial effect is warming
3) Helps decrease the production of *ama* (toxins)

Recipe:

1 Tbsp	lime juice
1/3 cup	orange juice
¾ cup	chopped peeled ginger root
½ cup	raisins

Combine ingredients and chop to desired texture by
hand or in food processor.

Lassi

Lassi is a refreshing drink made from yogurt that can be taken with meals to aid in digestion. It is best made from fresh yogurt. This drink is the natural way to get acidophilus in the diet and improve colon health. It is a great source of vitamin B12.

Plain Lassi:
Put 1 part yogurt into blender with 3, 4, or 5 parts water according to preference. (More water makes the lassi lighter and easier to digest.) Blend for 60 seconds. Remove any foam that forms on the top from the blending process.

Digestive Lassi:
Mix ½ cup yogurt, 2 cups room-temperature water, ¼ tsp ground cumin, ¼ tsp salt in blender for 60 seconds. Skim foam off top. Makes enough for two large glasses.

Sweet Lassi:
Mix ½ cup yogurt, 2 cups room-temperature water, ½ tsp turbinado sugar, 4 drops rose water, ¼ tsp cardamom in blender for 60 seconds. Skim foam off top. Makes enough for two large glasses.

Moong Dahl

Moong dahl (sometimes spelled "mung") is a split bean and the most digestible of the legumes. Moong beans are green, but when they have been dehulled and split they look like tiny split peas — yellow in color.

Plain beans are bland – adding spices make them more exciting. Flavors are best carried in lipid or fats (oils).

Ingredients:

½ cup	moong beans
1 ½ cups	water
¼ tsp	turmeric powder
½ tsp	coriander powder
½ tsp	cumin seeds
¼ tsp	salt
1 tsp	ghee (clarified butter) or olive oil
8 Leaves	fresh cilantro

Method:
- Rinse beans several times until no foam appears.
- Place beans in water and bring to boil.
- Turn down to a simmer.
- Remove any scum or foam that appears on top of water.
- Cook for 60 minutes.
- In a small frying pan, add oil and cumin seeds. When the seeds start to fry, turn down heat and add the rest of spices, stirring so that they do not burn.
- Mix thoroughly into beans.
- Garnish with chopped fresh cilantro leaves.

Pineapple Chutney

Pineapple chutney is pitta pacifying. It is sweet and mild.

Ingredients:

1 cup	fresh pineapple cubed
2 tsp	ghee
¼ tsp	cumin seed
1/8 tsp	turmeric
¼ tsp	cinnamon
1 Tbsp	turbinado sugar
1 pinch	salt

Method:

- Sauté cumin in ghee.
- Add pineapple and all other ingredients
- Simmer for 10-15 minutes.
- Let cool for 20 minutes and serve.

Stewed Apples

Use organic apples whenever possible. Stewed apples provides lively *prana*, and taken first thing in the morning helps to awaken the digestive fire (called *agni*) making digestion more complete throughout the rest of the day. Pears can also be prepared this way. Apples may be stewed using a quick method or a slow method:

Quick Method (Single Serving)
1. Peel and core 1 ripe apple.
2. Slice into small pieces, and place in pot.
3. Add ¼ cup spring water.
4. Add 2 whole cloves.
5. Cover pot and boil for 5 minutes.
6. Remove cloves and serve.

Slow Method (Single Serving)
1. Peel and core 1 ripe apple.
2. Slice into small pieces, and place in pot.
3. Add ¼ cup spring water.
3. Add 5 whole cloves.
4. Cover pot and cook for 20-30 minutes on low heat.

OR

Place ingredients in crockpot on high and cook for 1 hour.

5. Remove cloves and serve.

Spice Water

Drink all day long until 6 P.M. during purification diet.

Boil 1 quart of spring water for 5 minutes. Pour into a thermos. Add the following spices in WHOLE seed form:

¼ tsp cumin seeds
¼ tsp coriander seeds
½ tsp fennel seeds

Sip the spice water throughout the day every half hour or so. You may drink other water during the day according to thirst, but try to drink all the spice water by 6 P.M. Drinking the spice water after 6 P.M. may keep you awake at night due to its diuretic effect.

Spice water must be made fresh every day.

Swiss Chard

Use:
An important addition to other vegetables taken with a main meal.

Why:
1) Supplies both bitter and astringent tastes
2) A wonderful source of vitamins and minerals
3) An excellent source of fresh, high-prana food

Ingredients:
1 package of fresh Swiss chard (approximately 1 lb.)
1 lemon
Sprinkle of salt

Preparation:
Be sure to wash the leaves thoroughly. Some people prefer to cut the leaves off the central stem discarding the stem or using it for soups. Place in large pot with vegetable steamer and water. Steam for approximately 10-15 minutes. Serve with a squeeze of lemon juice and a sprinkle of salt.

Comment:
Chard cooks down to almost nothing. A full pot of chard will reduce to a very small proportion. One package is easily consumed by two people.

Unleavened Bread

Unleavened bread is made immediately after mixing the flour and water without having to wait for the bread to rise.

Ingredients:

½ tsp   salt
2/3 cups   whole-wheat pastry flour
1 2/3 cups   unbleached white flour
2 tsp   olive oil or ghee (clarified butter)
½ cup   water

Method:

Mix ingredients together and knead with hands. Pinch off a golf-ball-sized piece of dough, and form it into a ball. Roll it into a round ball using a rolling pin on a floured surface. When all of the dough balls have been rolled out, dry fry them individually. (No oil is used.) A cast-iron skillet works best for this purpose. Put the skillet on medium to high heat. The bread will tend to puff up or form little bubbles – when they appear, flip bread over. Cooking takes only a minute or two.

When done, you may spread a few drops of ghee over the top.

Yogurt

Procedure:
1. Bring 1 cup milk to a boil in a small pot.
2. Let the milk cool to a hot bathwater temperature (less than 120 degrees Fahrenheit — 108 degrees is ideal.) Put your hand on the side of the pot to test the temperature. If you can just barely hold your hand on the side, it is about the right temperature. (This usually takes 12-15 minutes depending on the amount of milk and the amount of heat your pot holds.)
3. Place warm milk in a wide-mouth thermos.
4. Add ½ tsp plain yogurt from the store and stir.
5. Leave mixture undisturbed for 8 hours.
6. *Note:* If you make yogurt before retiring, it may be left at room temperature until it is eaten at lunch. Do not refrigerate, unless you are saving some for starter for your next batch. Consume yogurt on the day it is made. Yogurt is best when it is fresh, not old and sour.

Appendix III

Resources

AYURVEDIC EDUCATION AND TRAINING

New World Ayurveda
1522 State St.
Santa Barbara, CA 93101
www.newworldayurveda.com
Email: newworldayurveda@yahoo.com
888-833-2108

MEDITATION TRAINING

Natural Meditation
New World Ayurveda
1522 State St.
Santa Barbara, CA 93101
www.newworldayurveda.com
Email: newworldayurveda@yahoo.com
888-833-2108

Transcendental Meditation
www.tm.org

Primordial Sound Meditation
www.chopra.com

Art of Living Meditation
www.artofliving.org